HIV-AIDS

In India and Developing Countries

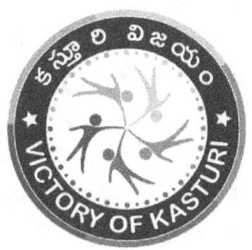

Dr. Yanamadala Murali Krishna, MD

ALL RIGHTS RESERVED

All rights reserved. No part of this publication may be reproduced, stored in or introduced into a retrieval system, or transmitted, in any form by any means may it be electronically, mechanical, optical, chemical, manual, photocopying, or recording without prior written permission of the Publisher/ Author.

HIV-AIDS
In India and Developing Countries
of
Dr. Yanamadala Murali Krishna, MD

Lakshmi Vaidyasala
Central Bank of India,
Current Account: 3732310770
IFSC Code: CBIN0283363
Phone Pe / Google Pay 9491031492

Dr. Yanamadala Murali Krishna,
4-50, Main Road, Indrapalem,
Kakinada – 533006, Andhra Pradesh, India
peopleagainstaids@yahoo.co.in
Ph:
E-mail: peopleagainstaids@yahoo.co.in

© Dr. Yanamadala Murali Krishna, MD

ISBN (Paperback): 978-81-969150-7-0

Published By: Kasturi Vijayam
Published on: May-2024

Print On Demand

Ph:0091-9515054998
Email: Kasturivijayam@gmail.com
Book Available
@
Amazon (Worldwide), flipkart

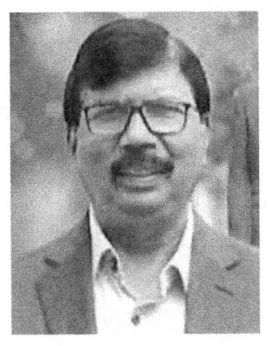

Dr. K. Babji, MS, MCh (Neuro)

Vice Chancellor

Dr YSR University of Health Sciences,

Vijayawada 520008,

Andhra Pradesh, India

Insightful Perspective from a Developing Country

I am very glad to go through the book written by Dr. Yanamadala Murali Krishna. The origin of HIV infection, its discovery, and the Nobel Prize winnings for the discovery were nicely illustrated. I remember my days at JIPMER in 1985 as a Senior Resident when I published my first article on HIV in a journal club. The architecture and epidemiology of HIV infection were effectively elaborated. The sources and ways of spread were dealt with very well, and the ways to prevent further spread were clearly explained.

I remember the days when we as surgeons were so much worried and panicked about HIV and AIDS. The disease has been controlled so well by the government, and now HIV and AIDS have become routine diseases. The Indian outlook, its treatment in different stages, and its success were also narrated very well. The association between HIV & TB, pregnancy, and other diseases was also discussed in this book. Life with HIV, once thought to be miserable, is now made as normal as possible, provided those with HIV take the necessary precautions.

Dr. Murali Krishna has discussed the vaccine against HIV and its issues so nicely, and he has mentioned how healthcare workers are advised to take universal healthcare precautions.

I am sure this book is good not only for the general public but also for doctors who are not closely related to HIV patients. I wish Dr. Yanamadala Murali Krishna great success in his future endeavours.

HIV is all around us!

For more than four decades, AIDS has plagued the world, especially in developing and poor countries. With all the catalysts contributing to the spread of this disease in our society, it is even more difficult to keep it at bay. There is no other pandemic in world history that has lasted so long. Moreover, HIV is an infection for life. In the present context, where it is no longer a major problem for developed countries, HIV has ceased to be a priority, and not many AIDS-related programs and research are going on. Consequently, there are fewer public health and awareness programs.

Neglect and complacency toward the issue are among the key factors contributing to the spread of HIV. With the ubiquitous presence of electronic gadgets, there is a constant stimulus for sexual activity for those entering youth. In such a situation, youth need to be more aware of HIV, which primarily spreads through sexual contact. HIV infection remains dormant for about a decade before surfacing as AIDS. As a result, it continues to spread without the knowledge of both partners.

HIV differs from other infectious diseases in that it does not spread through air or insects. Sexual contact with infected individuals transmits HIV. Only through awareness and preventive measures can we control the spread of this disease

As a 23-year full-time AIDS medical specialist with extensive study and experience caring for a large number of patients, it is my social obligation to author this book. Developing countries only follow the topics and issues addressed in HIV/AIDS books written by developed countries. This book covers a multitude of issues that no other book can match. I have tried to make complex science topics as easy to understand as possible. However, in developing countries, the course and presentation of the disease are different from those in developed countries. This book is the perception of a physician from a developing country, and I hope it serves as an informative read for the general public and a valuable resource for health care workers in third-world countries.

Despite the availability of effective antiretroviral therapy (ART), our patients do not have the same relief, normal life, or life expectancy as those in industrialized countries. The lack of specialized AIDS experts and the inability to recognize new issues not discussed in books, primarily by western authors, are contributing factors. However, I believe that I have largely overcome this obstacle, thanks to the support of my satisfied patients. My patients have given me more insights about this disease than the books I studied.

Sex, a basic instinct like eating and sleeping, primarily transmits HIV, the virus that causes AIDS. Children who constantly grow up and enter adulthood may have casual sex. There is a constant need for education about HIV. To fulfil such a big responsibility, this book should be a handy tool to educate the public, healthcare workers, and HIV patients.

-Dr. Yanamadala Murali Krishna, MD

Acknowledgements

Kudos to my wife, Yanamadala Geetha, who went through each chapter of this book in Telugu multiple times and provided suggestions for clarity. Thanks to my son Ramakrishna, who not only designed the cover page but also offered guidance on many technical aspects. I am grateful to my friend and humanist, Mr. Penmetsa Subbaraju, who spent a significant amount of money to support a clinic for HIV patients in Palakollu and encouraged me to write this book. I am grateful to Mr. Chandrasekhar Konda of the Rural Hope Foundation (USA), Mr. Siva Annapureddy, Dr. Jana Veerabhadra Prasad, and others for their generous contribution towards the publication of this book. Many thanks to my friends, Mr. Bollareddy Sridhar Reddy, and Mr. Kudupudi Nageswara Rao, for making the necessary pictures presentable.

-Dr. Yanamadala Murali Krishna, MD

Research is to see what everybody else has seen, and to think what nobody else has thought.

Albert Szent-Gyorgyi,
Nobel Laureate in Physiology or Medicine, 1937

Contents

1. The Beginning of AIDS 1
2. The Origins and Journey of HIV 5
3. Human Immunodeficiency Virus 10
4. Global impact of AIDS 20
5. Routes of HIV infection 25
6. HIV Prevention Methods 31
7. The ravage of AIDS 37
8. AIDS: The Indian scenario 40
9. HIV-AIDS 45
10. HIV - AIDS Testing 50
11. Treatment of HIV - AIDS 55
12. Two-Drug Antiretroviral Therapy 63
13. Fight for the Rights of AIDS-Affected 66
14. HIV and Tuberculosis 71
15. Tuberculin response to assess AIDS severity in HIV- TB patients 78
16. HIV and Pregnancy 82
17. Living with HIV 86
18. HIV Cure Research 90
19. The Promise and challenge of an AIDS Vaccine 97
20. AIDS impact on women and Children 102
21. HIV and Medical profession 105
22. HIV and Skin diseases 108
23. UNAIDS and other Global organizations' fight against AIDS 111
24. Indian Generics and Global HIV Treatment Equity 114
Dr. Yanamadala Murali Krishna: A Champion in Public Health 118

1. The Beginning of AIDS

A new disease was identified in the United States by observing unusual clusters of rare diseases that occurred exclusively in immunocompromised patients.

All developed countries regularly collect information about the health of their people and diseases that occur in the country. The US Department of Health and Human Services publishes a weekly newsletter called the 'Morbidity and Mortality Weekly Report' (MMWR), which contains data collected by the US Centers for Disease Control and Prevention (CDC). Primarily read by doctors and public health personnel, this newsletter publishes scientific information, statistics, and background information on diseases.

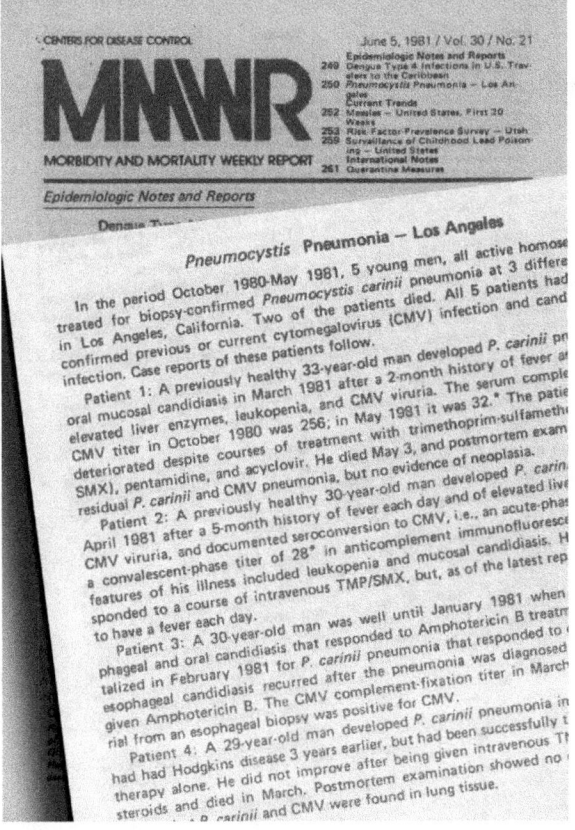

The June 5, 1981, issue of MMWR brought to the attention of doctors five gay men (male homosexuals—'gays") from Los Angeles who contracted the extremely rare fungus infection of the lungs, *Pneumocystis carinii* (now called *Pneumocystis jiroveci*).

Pneumocystis is usually present in the environment and rarely causes disease in patients lacking functional immune systems.

A rare skin cancer called 'Kaposi's sarcoma' was also observed in some other gay people within the next month. Both diseases are seen rarely in genetic disorders where the immune system is almost completely deficient or in situations where the immunity is severely damaged due to leukaemia (blood cancer), cancer treatment, or organ transplant therapy. These diseases, seen only in one person every few years, when presented in clusters, have made doctors think that they are dealing with a new immunodeficient disease.

The Stigma of AIDS: Misconceptions & Marginalization

In the early days of this immune-afflicting disease, it was diagnosed primarily in gay men and called 'Gay Related Immune Deficiency' (GRID). The disease was also known as slim disease, as they were severely wasted. Later, researchers identified the disease in several other groups. So, the four 'H's were considered risk factors for the disease. They were homosexuals, haemophiliacs, heroin (injection drug users), and Haitians. This derogatory categorization was the source of contempt for those belonging to those groups. There was extreme fear and stigma towards them in society.

Human societies often shun those suffering from severe wasting diseases at a young age. Those afflicted with this newly identified disease suffer from a variety of ailments and die in a matter of weeks or months. Due to the disdain for gays in society and not knowing how this disorder spreads, everyone in society, including those in the medical field, used to keep those patients away with intense fear and hallucinations. In the early days, hospital personnel wore personal protective equipment (PPE kits), much like astronauts, to dispose of the bodies of people who died of this disorder.

Due to the lack of access to medical care for those suffering from this disease, the patients had to provide palliative care to one another. These patients suffered a lot in the early years because of the overwhelming publicity and exaggerations. Many rare infections affect patients with this disease. We refer to these as opportunistic infections. Microbial organisms that would not cause disease in the general population can cause disease in them, taking advantage of the weakened immune system. These patients present with extreme weight loss, rare pneumonia, rare cancers, an unrelenting fever, and constant diarrhoea. Also, there are various sores and boils on the body and mouth. These looked like moving skeletons.

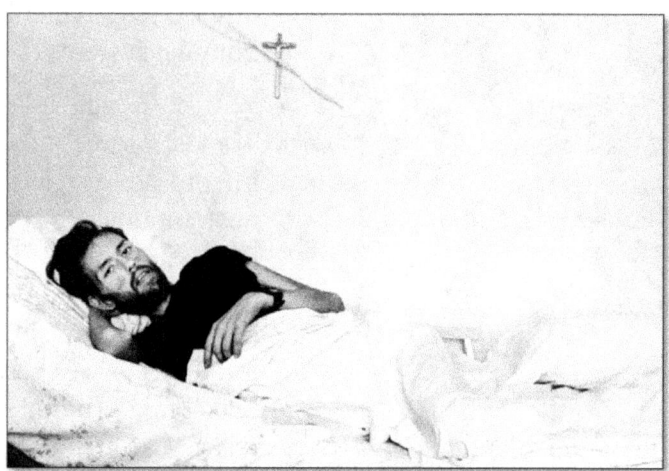

In May 1990, David Kirby was in the final stages of AIDS. He was an outspoken activist, and this haunting photo humanized the struggles of those battling the disease during the crisis.

HIV-AIDS

Unveiling the Culprit: Identifying the Cause of AIDS

Genetic disorders causing a total lack of immunity are called 'Primary Immunodeficiency Syndromes'. Children suffering from such primary immunodeficiency syndromes usually suffer from severe multiple infections in infancy and die before reaching adolescence. But the 'gays' who are affected by such diseases are not children but young adults. They were found to have no genetic defects or other causes that seriously weaken the immune system. Realizing that they were infected with a new disease that destroys the immune system, they started calling it 'acquired immunodeficiency syndrome' or 'AIDS' in September 1982. Expanding on the acronym 'AIDS, 'Acquired means acquired during life rather than at birth; Immune means immunity; Deficiency means decrease; a Syndrome is a set of symptoms. AIDS can be called an 'infectious disease that destroys immunity.' However, a deeper search of this disease revealed that reports of cases with similar symptoms date back several decades. Among those who suffer from this type of immunodeficient disease are those who inject drugs with contaminated needles, gay people, haemophiliacs, those who have received blood transfusions on various occasions, sexual partners of the previous groups, and their children who were infected.

Dispelling Fears and Clarifying Risks:

However, the Centers for Disease Control declared in 1982 that only sexual contact, injections, and blood transfusions could transmit the disease from one person to another. This announcement has, to some extent, changed the fear of spreading the infection from the infected people through the air, touching them, using spoons, plates, glasses, bathrooms or commodes, and insects like mosquitoes. However, after knowing that this disease is spread through sex and drug injections, people used to dismiss these patients as strays. In the early years, even politicians did not talk about this disease. This resulted in a lack of adequate funding for research into the disease. Due to this, there was not much awareness and caution about AIDS. HIV tests became available four years later, in 1985.

Early Champions in AIDS Research and Advocacy:

Dr. Michael Gottlieb first identified *Pneumocystis* pneumonia in gay men. The Centers for Disease Control and Prevention investigated the rare *Pneumocystis* pneumonia, revealing that the disease had only affected one patient in the past 15 years. Kaposi's sarcoma is a rare blood vessel cancer in the elderly, especially in the skin. Dermatologists Dr. Alvin Freedman-Keene and Dr. Linda Laubenstein were the first to notice Kaposi's sarcoma in young gay men.

Dr. Gerald Friedland, a physician in the Bronx area of New York City, first reported AIDS among drug users. At that time, those who took injection drugs used to rent needles in areas called shooting galleries and go for injections. Shooting gallery operators used to rent the same syringes to one another without cleaning them. Because of this, the virus that caused AIDS spread very rapidly among them.

Dr. James Oleski, a paediatrician at Beth Israel Medical Center in Newark, New Jersey, was the first to diagnose AIDS in children.

Dr. Margaret Fischl of the University of Miami diagnosed *Pneumocystis* pneumonia and Kaposi's sarcoma in Haitian male and female patients. Dr. Rosabend also noted that AIDS is spreading not only among gay people but also between male and female couples. Three of the first seven patients identified in July 1981 by Dr. Rosen Baum of France were women.

In July 1982, the US Centers for Disease Control announced that two haemophiliacs who had taken factor VIII had contracted AIDS.

As the AIDS disease was detected not only among homosexuals—those who took injection drugs—but also among children, women, and heterosexual men, it was understood that it was a scourge of the whole society. However, due to the demonstrations and struggles demanding the rights of AIDS, patients were mostly from the gay community; political elites and the public also considered it a gay disease for a long time.

AIDS in Africa: Recognizing a Pre-Existing Epidemic

In October 1983, a CDC team led by Dr. Joe McCormick visited hospitals in Kinshasa, Congo. They identified dozens of people suffering from AIDS symptoms in the hospitals, concluding that AIDS was already prevalent in Africa. Since the 1960s, it has been known that some people were dying of a mysterious disease in the towns of Central Africa.

By the time AIDS was first diagnosed in America, it was estimated that 250,000 people were infected with the virus that causes the disease. Researchers later estimated that millions of people had already contracted the virus before the first diagnosis of AIDS in Africa.

2. The Origins and Journey of HIV

HIV, transmitted from chimpanzees and gorillas to humans, spread rapidly through urbanization, colonization, war, and medical interventions.

Identifying the Culprit: The Discovery of HIV

Within a short while after the identification of AIDS in America, a similar illness was detected in African countries and European countries. Initially referred to as 'Gay Related Immune Deficiency' (GRID), 'Slim Disease', 'Gay Cancer', 'Gay Plague', and so on, 'AIDS' (acquired immunodeficiency syndrome) became the official name in 1982. In 1983, researchers identified the virus that causes this disease. Later research showed that the origins of this virus were in Africa.

By December 1982, Dr. Willy Rosenbaum of the Claude Bernard Hospital in Paris, the capital of France, had diagnosed AIDS in 29 patients. Dr. Willy Rosenbaum sent a lymph node sample from a 33-year-old patient to the Pasteur Institute in Paris for further investigation. In 1983, medical researchers Luc Montagnier and François Barre Sinoussi of the Pasteur Institute isolated the virus from the lymph node. In April 1984, American medical researcher Robert Gallo announced that he had identified the virus. Initially, it was called Lymphadenopathy Associated Virus (LAV) and Human T cell Lymphotropic Virus III (HTLV III). By identifying the virus and growing it in cell culture in the laboratory, scientists developed tests to confirm HIV by 1985. Identifying the virus also helped develop drugs to treat HIV infection. Virologists named this virus 'Human Immunodeficiency Virus' (HIV) in 1986. In 2008, 25 years after the discovery of this virus, Dr. Luc Montagnier and Dr. Françoise Barre Sinoussi were awarded the Nobel Prize in Medicine/Physiology.

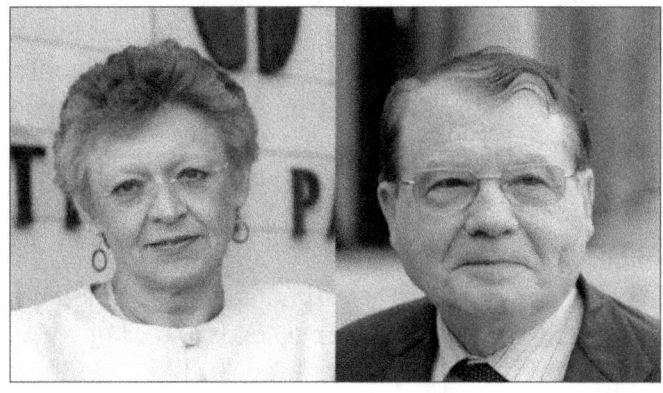

Dr. Françoise Barre Sinoussi   *Dr. Luc Montagnier*

HIV's Origin in African Non-human Primates:

Significant advancements in genetic engineering enabled the creation of a comprehensive genetic map of virus samples. With this type of mapping, it was recognized that large numbers of people in Africa had been infected with HIV for a long time. Researchers discovered significant similarities between the genes of HIV, which causes AIDS, and the genes of the 'Simian Immunodeficiency Virus' (SIV), which infects chimpanzees in African countries.

Viruses that cause many diseases are transmitted from animals to humans. These are called zoonoses. Some of these viruses later become transmissible between humans. Extensive research has shown that the Human Immunodeficiency Virus, which causes AIDS, also 'jumped' from animals to humans.

Early Spread: Urbanization, Colonization, and Sex Trade

In the 19th century, many European countries invaded the poorest African countries, making them their colonies. They built railways, cities, roads, and bridges in the respective African countries for trade and transportation. Belgium occupied the then region of Zaire, now known as the 'Democratic Republic of Congo'. At that time, it was called 'Belgian Congo'. Belgium developed a small town called Leopoldville into a big city. As a part of large-scale urbanization, many men from rural areas of the country migrated to urban areas to work on constructing railways, roads, and buildings. Under such circumstances, commercial sex inevitably flourished, and brothels grew rampant. Along with that, venereal diseases became rampant.

The Allied Powers attacked Cameroon, a colony of the Central Powers, from five sides during the First World War. The Allied Powers that attacked Cameroon from the southeast included 1,000 French Congolese troops, 600 Belgian Congolese troops, and one hundred French and ten Belgian military officers. The soldiers were from African countries, and the officers were from Europe. They all reached the Mulundu region of Cameroon in late 1914 via the Congo River, a tributary of the Sangha. However, there was not much resistance from the German army. In no time, the food reserves they had brought were empty. Food supplies had to come from the far-off region of Brazzaville. Many soldiers used to go into the forest to hunt chimpanzees and gorillas from the nearby forest for food. During the hunting and butchering of gorillas for their meat, someone in the army contracted the 'Simian Immunodeficiency Virus.' Many African tribes also hunt chimpanzees and gorillas in nearby forests for meat. Then, in mid-1916, the army reached Leopoldville (present-day Kinshasa) in the Belgian Congo. In Leopoldville, it spread from soldiers to sex workers. So, 'Patient Zero'*—the first patient was from Congo. Leopoldville, which had a population of 14,000 at that time, crossed 200,000 in three and a half decades. By 1950, it is estimated that around 500 people would be infected with HIV. In the 1950s, a traditional sex worker known as a free woman in Leopoldville had three or four regular clients a year. As a result of the migration of men to work in construction projects, from rural areas to cities, commercial sex work also increased exponentially. With the migration, each sex worker used to get three or four visitors a night. Since then, the spread of HIV had been rampant.

In 1959, the University of Washington in the United States collected 1213 blood samples in Zaire for malaria research. In 1998, University of Washington researchers found HIV antibodies in one of those samples. Researchers identified the Bantu man as ZR59, marking this as the earliest case of HIV. In 1960, researchers discovered HIV in the lymph node of a woman who had died from lymphoma cancer. This patient is named DRC 60.

From SIV to HIV: The Zoonotic Crossover

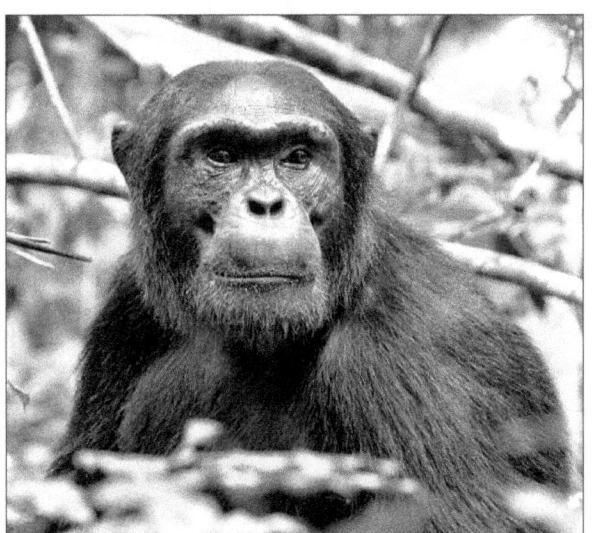

Simian Immunodeficiency Virus (SIVcpz), which infects chimpanzees (scientific name *'Pan troglodytes troglodytes'*), causes an AIDS-like disease in them. Dr. Beatrice Hahn of the University of Pennsylvania isolated mitochondria from more than 7,000 stool and urine samples collected from chimpanzees and gorillas in Cameroon and mapped the genes of the 'Simian Immunodeficiency Virus' in them. These findings confirmed the origin of HIV. From these SIVcpz, HIV-1 originated. A rare type of HIV, HIV-2, had been identified as being transmitted to humans from the sooty mangabey (scientific name: *Sarcocebus ates*) virus SIVsm. HIV-1 group O is derived from the Simian Immunodeficiency Virus SIVgor that infects gorillas. It was learned that some of the chimpanzees nurtured by wildlife conservationist Jane Goodall were infected with SIV and died of the disease.

The Simian Immunodeficiency Virus was transmitted from chimpanzees, gorillas, and monkeys to humans through hunting and butchering of meat in the forests of Cameroon. From there, it reached Kinshasa via the Congo River, the only long-distance transport route at the time. French researcher Jacques Pepe recognized this journey of HIV. Almost all variants of HIV had been identified as having originated in the country of Cameroon.

HIV, which has been wreaking havoc for over 40 years, belongs to the genus Lentivirus of the Retroviridae family. Lenti means slow, sluggish. meaning that this virus causes disease very slowly and over a prolonged period of time. As the infected person is symptom-free for a lengthy period, the virus would be passed on to more people through sexual contact. Shortly after AIDS surfaced in the US, it was identified that the disease had already spread rampantly in African countries. HIV tests conducted in the early years of AIDS among sex workers in some cities of Central and West Africa revealed that 90% of them were infected with the virus.

The Simian Immunodeficiency Virus, which had been infiltrating African populations since the beginning of the 20th century, had transformed into the Human Immunodeficiency Virus by 1921 and was spreading without any symptoms.

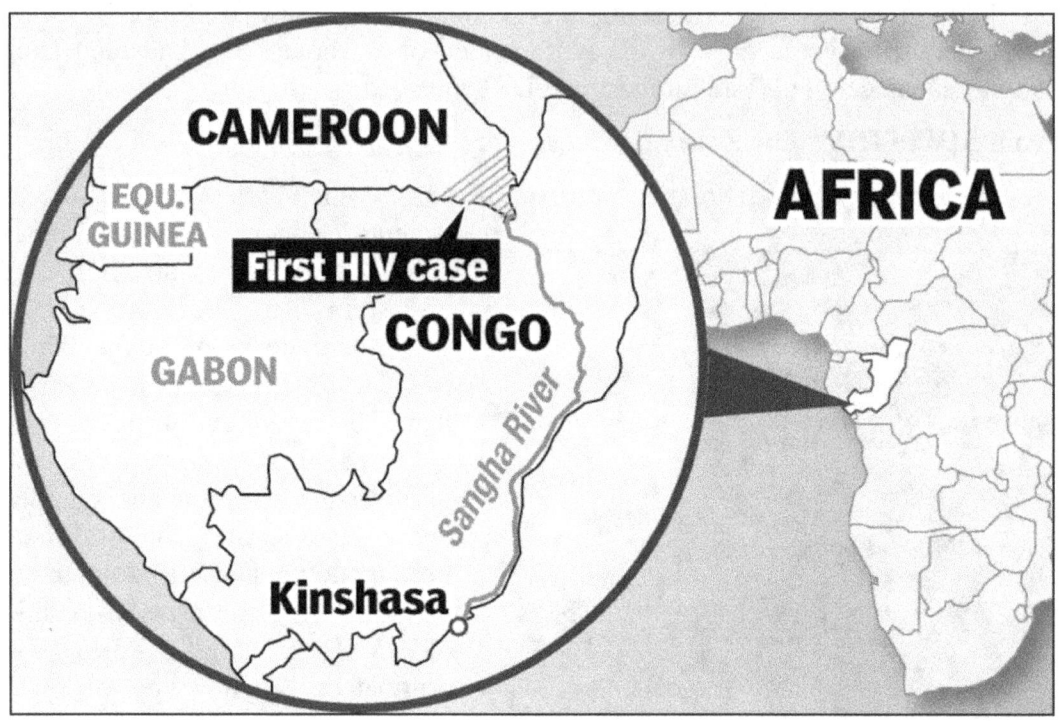

The early spread of HIV is thought to have followed the Sangha River from its origins in southeastern Cameroon into Kinshasa (formerly known as Léopoldville), the capital of the Democratic Republic of Congo, before extending further

As the sex trade was so prevalent, sexually transmitted diseases spread rampantly. Sex workers and men infected by them used to queue up at clinics conducted by Belgian doctors. Those doctors used to give their patients the newly available penicillin and other injections. Back then, there was no practice of cleaning syringes. They used to give injections with the same syringe to many the patients who visited them. Since the 1950s, doctors and medical staff thought syringes could be contaminated and started cleaning syringes by boiling and flushing them. HIV, which entered society from chimpanzees and gorillas in the forest, spread widely among the people of Congo and Cameroon due to these issues.

From 1921 to 1959, Belgian authorities administered injection drugs as part of large-scale public health measures for treatment of malaria, African trypanosomiasis, and leprosy. HTLV1, and Hepatitis C viruses Some researchers believe that the large-scale smallpox vaccination at the time also contributed to the spread of HIV in those communities.

Global Expansion: From Africa to Haiti and Beyond

In 1960, when the Congolese people revolted and gained independence, the Belgian doctors left the country. The United Nations sent about 4,500 professionals, including doctors, teachers, and others from various countries, to provide medical, educational, and other services to the Congolese people. It is believed that some of these professionals may have unknowingly carried HIV from the Congo to Haiti during 1967–68. At the time, Haiti was a destination for sex tourism, and there was a trade in blood products. The United States used to import blood from Haiti to treat bleeding disorders like haemophilia and other conditions. This is how HIV is thought to have entered the American bloodline. HIV then spread to cities like Los Angeles, New York, and San Francisco through sexual transmission, particularly among gay men who had visited Haiti, which is geographically close to the United States. Later, it spread across the country.

It is a sad truth that HIV spread from non-human primates to humans in the early days due to urbanization, imperialism, war, and well-intentioned public health measures.

*The book 'And the Band Played On' by Randy Shilts portrayed Canadian flight attendant Gaetan Dugas as 'Patient Zero', who infected numerous people with HIV. However, he was not the first HIV patient. It is inaccurate to claim that HIV spread around the world because of him. Dugas received a diagnosis of Kaposi's sarcoma in 1980 and passed away in 1984. The author Randy Shilts mistakenly identified 'Patient O' (O for 'Outside of California') as 'Zero' (0) in the flow chart created by the US Centers for Disease Control to identify the spread of AIDS.

3. Human Immunodeficiency Virus

HIV, which is roughly one hundred-millionth of a metre in spherical shape, has many unique characteristics that make it a major challenge for the world.

Viruses are the bridge between living and non-living matter, in the process of life arising from non-living matter. The virus cannot strive on its own. Viruses are made up of certain chemicals. Once they enter distinct species, they develop making use of mechanism of the respective species (host).

Viral Structure:

The genetic information of all organisms is contained in two strands of DNA (double stranded DNA). The genetic information in viruses is carried in DNA or RNA. Some viruses contain this information in a single strand rather than in two strands (double-stranded).

The human immunodeficiency virus (HIV) has a spherical or cone-shaped core surrounded by a lipid membrane envelope. The virus particle is approximately 120 nanometres (nm) in diameter. The inner core, or nucleocapsid, contains two copies of single-stranded, positive-sense RNA strands, along with the enzyme's reverse transcriptase, integrase, and protease. The HIV genome consists of 9 genes and is approximately 9.7 kilobases (kb) in length. The nucleocapsid is surrounded by a matrix protein, which gives the virus its distinct cone-shaped core. The matrix protein is enclosed by a lipid bilayer envelope derived from the host cell membrane.

The thorn-like large structures of the HIV virus that protrude from the envelope are known as glycoprotein 120 (gp120). A small transmembrane glycoprotein (gp41) is the continuation part of the envelope from gp120 to the inside. It is through this glycoprotein 120 that the virus attaches to the CD4+ protein on human cells and enters the cells of the human body.

Reverse Transcription: A Unique Replication Strategy

The human immunodeficiency virus (HIV) belongs to the genus Lentivirus of the family Retroviridae. Retroviruses are named for an enzyme called reverse transcriptase. This enzyme, present in retroviruses, converts the RNA in the virus into DNA. The formation of DNA from RNA with this reverse transcriptase enzyme was a new discovery that was not known until the 1960s. Until then, only the transcription of DNA to RNA was known to biologists. David Baltimore and Howard Temin were awarded the Nobel Prize in 1975 for discovering this 'reverse transcription' process. The DNA made in this way can integrate and become part of the genome of the human or respective host organism. The Lentivirus genus is named because lentiviruses are slow progressing, very slow long-term pathogens.

Place of HIV in the Viral World

Retroviruses cause a variety of diseases in both animals and humans. Retroviruses can cause malignant cancers, autoimmune diseases, immunodeficiency syndromes, and aplastic and haemolytic anaemias. In fact, the human immunodeficiency virus (HIV) that causes AIDS is neither the first nor the last retrovirus to affect human evolution. Approximately 8% of the human genome is composed of human endogenous retroviruses (HERVs), remnants of ancient viral infections that have become a part of the human genome over millions of years of evolution. These HERVs are embedded in the human genome in a dormant state without causing any harm.

HIV Lifecycle: Infection, Replication, and Destruction:

HIV infection is initiated by attaching to a protein known as CD4+, which is present on the surface of some human cells. In the end, the virus sheds its envelope, and the nucleocapsid, which contains the viral genome and enzymes, enters the cell with the help of chemokine co-receptors called CCR5 and CXCR4. The HIV genome consists of nine genes.

Once inside the cell, the viral enzyme reverse transcriptase generates a DNA copy from the RNA of the virus. This viral DNA then becomes double-stranded, which is the same form as the human genome. This double-stranded viral DNA, called proviral DNA, then integrates into the human's DNA with the help of the viral enzyme integrase. Thus, the virus permanently becomes part of the human body, and the HIV infection persists for a lifetime. Consequently, the activation of HIV-infected CD4+ lymphocytes triggers the production of viral proteins.

The large viral protein molecules are cleaved by the viral enzyme protease to form complete virus particles (virions). These virions bud from the cell membrane of the CD4+ cell, enveloping themselves in the cell's membrane and releasing the virus particles.

HIV is a virus that attacks and destroys a specific type of cell in the body called CD4+ cells. These cells are a crucial part of the immune system and help fight off infections.

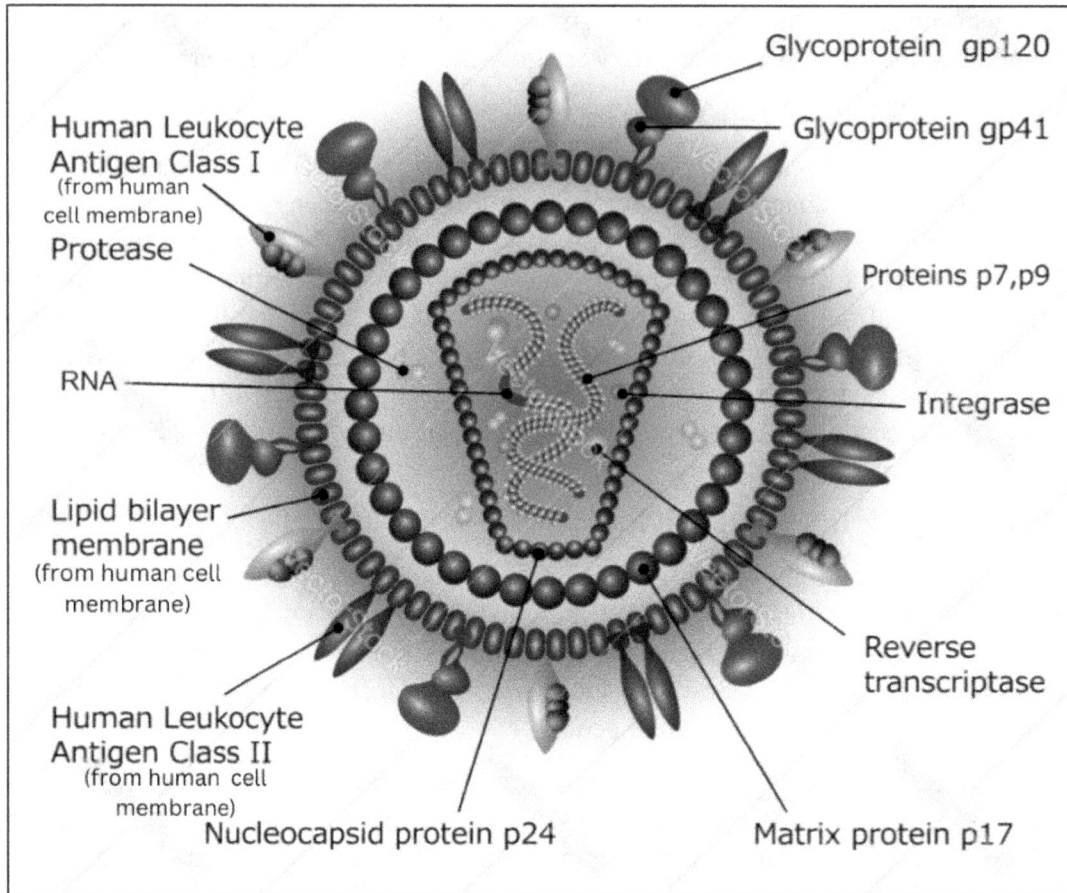

Structure of Human Immunodeficiency Virus

When HIV enters the body, it infects and takes over the CD4+ cells. Over time, the virus causes the CD4+ cells to die off through various processes, including programmed cell death (apoptosis), self-digestion (autophagy), and attacks by other immune cells called cytotoxic CD8 T cells.

As more CD4+ cells are destroyed, the immune system becomes weaker and less effective at fighting off diseases and infections. This decrease in CD4+ cells is a hallmark of HIV progression and the development of AIDS, which stands for acquired immunodeficiency syndrome.

HIV primarily infects cells that have a specific protein called CD4+ on their surface. These include helper T cells (a type of white blood cell), macrophages (cells that engulf and digest harmful substances), and Langerhans or Langerhans cells (cells that help activate other immune cells).

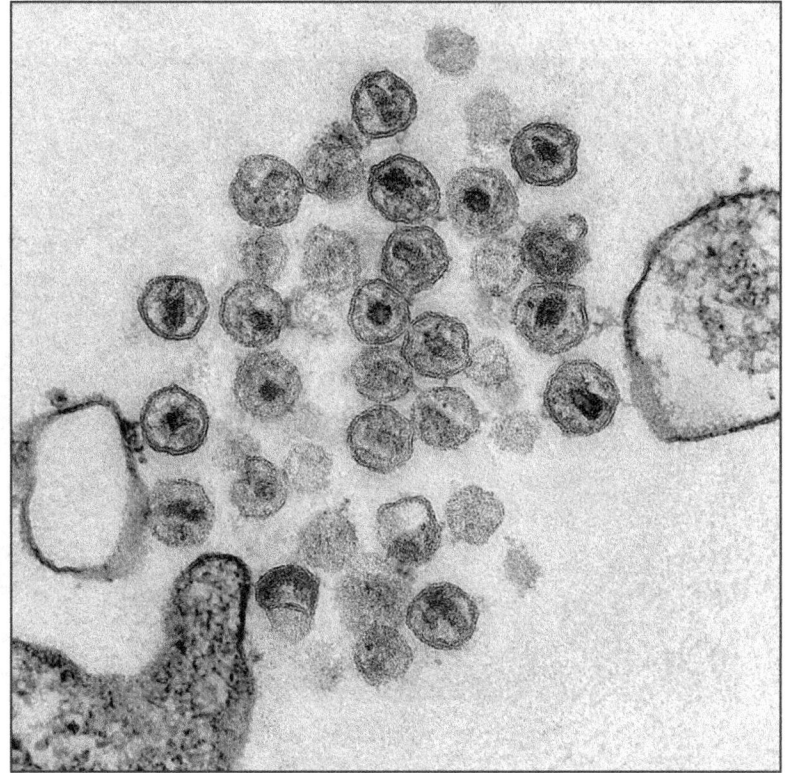

HIV Virion Particles Transmission Electron Micrograph

While the main way HIV enters the body is through sexual transmission involving a specific co-receptor called CCR5, HIV can also be transmitted through sharing needles among injecting drug users. In this case, another co-receptor called CXCR4 plays a role.

Once HIV infects helper T cells, it hijacks their machinery to produce more copies of the virus (called virions). Macrophages and Langerhans or Langerhans cells also serve as reservoirs for HIV, allowing the virus to replicate and spread further.

As more and more helper T cells are destroyed, the immune system becomes increasingly compromised and unable to defend against opportunistic infections, which are infections that take advantage of a weakened immune system. This susceptibility to opportunistic infections is a characteristic feature of AIDS.

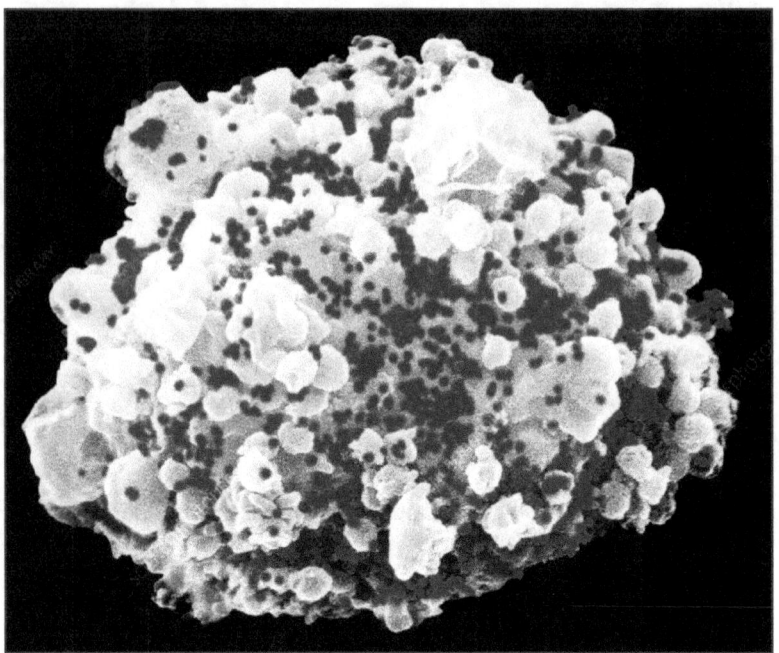

HIV virions being released from the CD4+ lymphocyte

In some HIV-infected macrophages, the virus remains latent without replicating. With the same dormancy mechanism, some CD4+ lymphocytes become memory cells. These memory cells can persist in the lymph nodes for a long time and act as a virus reservoir. Langerhans or Langerhans cells play a crucial role in the transmission of HIV from one person to another.

Macrophages, including microglia in the brain, Kupffer cells in the liver, and Langerhans cells in the skin, are crucial tissue-resident immune cells found in various organs. They play essential roles in immune surveillance, phagocytosis, and initiating innate immune responses within their respective tissues. However, upon encountering a pathogen like the HIV virus, it is primarily the dendritic cells (DCs), not macrophages, that migrate to nearby lymph nodes to initiate an adaptive immune response. DCs are specialized cells that present antigens to T cells in the lymph nodes. They do this quickly and effectively, initiating the adaptive immune response and activating T cells.

HIV (Human Immunodeficiency Virus) primarily infects a type of white blood cells called CD4+ lymphocytes, which play a crucial role in the body's immune system. However, HIV can only infect these cells when they are in an "activated" state.

Normally, only a small percentage (around 1%) of CD4+ lymphocytes are in an activated state at any given time. However, when the body is fighting an infectious disease, more CD4+ lymphocytes become activated to help combat the infection.

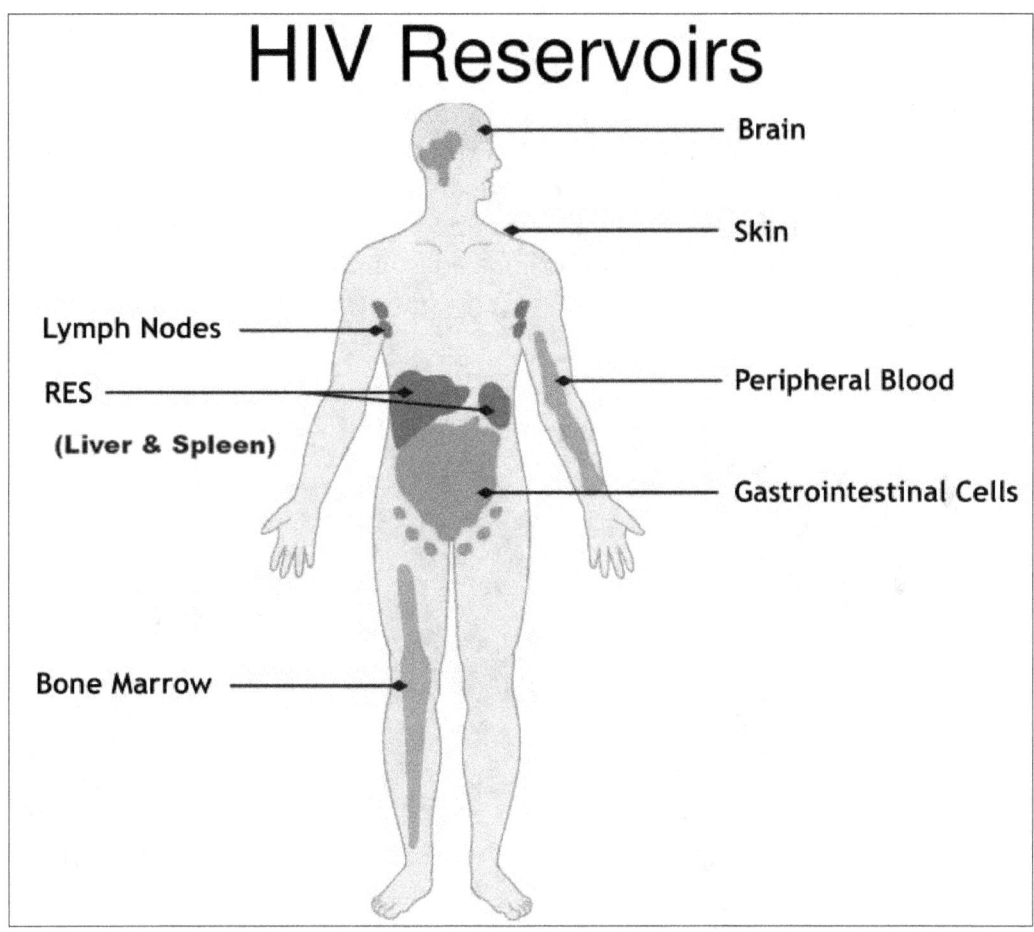

In people living with HIV, the proportion of activated CD4+ lymphocytes is higher than in other infectious diseases, ranging from 5% to 20%. During the initial acute stage of HIV infection, when the virus is first establishing itself in the body, the proportion of activated CD4+ lymphocytes can reach up to 50%.

This higher level of activated CD4+ lymphocytes in HIV-positive individuals provides more targets for the virus to infect and replicate, contributing to the gradual depletion of these crucial immune cells over time.

HIV Diversity: Different Types and Subtypes

There are two main types of HIV: HIV-1 and HIV-2. HIV-1 accounts for more than 99% of global HIV infections, while HIV-2 is mainly confined to West and Central Africa. Scientists first isolated HIV-1 in 1983 and HIV-2 in 1986. When referring to HIV without a type specified, it typically denotes HIV-1.

Both HIV-1 and HIV-2 can cause AIDS, but HIV-2 generally progresses more slowly. Transmission of HIV-2 from mother to child is also less common. Both HIV-1 and HIV-2 can infect an individual simultaneously. However, HIV-1 and HIV-2 are distinct types of the virus, not different stages of the same disease. HIV-1 does not evolve into HIV-2.

Four distinct cross-species transmission (crossover) events led to the evolution of HIV-1 from the simian immunodeficiency virus (SIV) in chimpanzees and gorillas, giving rise to the four groups: M (Main), O (Outlier), N (Non-M, Non-O), and P (Putative). The M group originated from SIV in chimpanzees and is responsible for the global AIDS pandemic. The O group originated from SIV in gorillas, while the N and P groups also originated from SIV in chimpanzees. The O, N, and P groups are relatively rare and largely confined to parts of Cameroon and neighbouring countries.

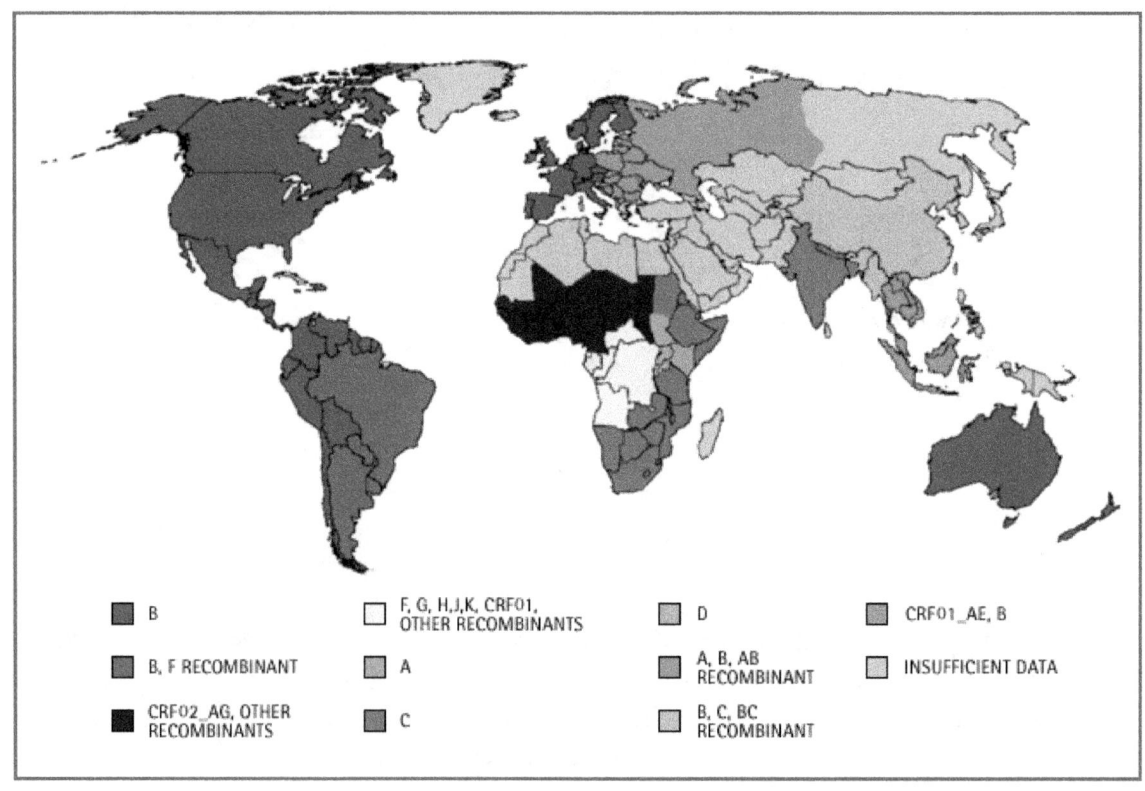

Global Distribution of HIV-1 Group M Clades

Group M is responsible for the global HIV pandemic, infecting over 80 million people and causing nearly 4 million deaths. HIV-1 group M has undergone significant genetic diversification within humans, with genetic differences ranging from 17% to 35%. These variants are known as clades or subtypes. HIV's high mutation rate is primarily due to errors in the activity of the viral reverse transcriptase enzyme during replication, resulting in vast genetic variation.

Nine major clades of HIV-1 group M have been identified: A, B, C, D, E, F, G, H, J, and K. Clade C accounts for approximately 50% of HIV-1 infections globally, while Clade B contributes about 12% and is primarily found in the Americas, Europe, and Asia. Additionally, researchers have identified over 100 circulating recombinant forms (CRFs) of HIV-1, resulting from recombination between different clades, with CRF02_AG being one of the most prevalent.

About 15000 people were infected with Group O, Group N was found in 20 people and Group P was identified in 2 people.

The genetic diversity of HIV-2 is very low. There are subtypes A to H. Subtypes A and B are more prevalent.

The protruding glycoprotein on the surface of the HIV-1 virion is gp120, and the structure that extends into the membrane is gp41, while in HIV-2, they are gp105 and gp36, respectively.

The Pace of HIV Progression: Disease Course

The human body typically produces detectable antibodies within a few weeks to three months following an HIV infection. Following the initial infection, there is a period of rapid viral replication, after which the virus establishes a chronic infection. Daily, an estimated 10 billion (10^{10}) HIV virions can be produced, potentially infecting millions to hundreds of millions (10^6 to 10^8) of CD4+ lymphocytes. However, due to the large production of blood cells, including CD4+ lymphocytes, in the bone marrow, the number of these lymphocytes decreases slowly. During the transcription of viral RNA into DNA by reverse transcriptase, a high number of errors occur, leading to a significant genetic mutation of HIV. These mutations can lead to viral variants with reduced infectivity or susceptibility to the immune response. Additionally, HIV can integrate its proviral DNA into the host genome, including less active regions like centromeres, establishing a latent reservoir. This reservoir contributes to persistent infection even with low levels of active viral replication.

Antiretroviral therapy (ART) can effectively suppress HIV replication, leading to a significant reduction in viral load and preventing new infections of cells. However, it does not eliminate the proviral DNA reservoir. Therefore, despite the high viral turnover during initial infection and the persistence of the viral reservoir, the number of CD4+ lymphocytes decreases slowly, especially in individuals receiving ART.

Once HIV enters the body, it infects specific cells, and there are two types of infection that can be established. In a productive (or active) HIV infection, the proviral DNA is integrated into the host cell's genome, and both viral RNA and proteins are produced, leading to the production of new viral particles, and eventually causing the death of the infected CD4+ T cells. As a result, the number of CD4+ T lymphocytes slowly decreases. Another type of infection is called a latent infection, which serves as a viral reservoir. In these latent cells, the proviral DNA remains integrated into the host cell's genome, but it does not actively produce viral RNA or proteins. The HIV proteins are also not produced, allowing these cells to survive for a long time without being recognized by the body's defence system (immune evasion).

Transition Between States:

HIV's ability to establish a latent reservoir within host cells poses a significant challenge to achieving complete eradication. While antiretroviral therapy (ART) effectively suppresses viral replication and allows individuals to live long and healthy lives, the virus persists in a low-level state within certain immune cells. This reservoir can be reactivated under various conditions, such as fluctuations in the immune system, inflammation, or the presence of other infections. Managing HIV, therefore, requires a multifaceted approach. Adherence to ART is crucial for controlling viral replication and minimizing the risk of reactivation. Additionally, lifestyle modifications that promote overall health, including stress management, sufficient sleep, and a balanced diet, contribute to a robust immune response and overall well-being.

The Challenge of Latency:

Latently infected cells form a hidden reservoir of HIV that persists even with effective antiretroviral therapy. This reservoir is a major obstacle to finding a cure for HIV, as these cells can reactivate and reignite the infection if treatment is stopped.

Understanding the dynamics of productive and latent HIV infections is crucial for developing effective treatment strategies and ultimately finding a cure for HIV/AIDS.

In some people with human lymphocyte antigen (HLA) types B57 and B27, the progression of HIV is slow. The infection progresses more rapidly in those with HLA B35 and B53.

The human immunodeficiency virus belongs to the retrovirus family. The lentivirus subclass includes HIV. 'Lenti' means slow, indicating that viruses in this subclass cause disease slowly over a long period of time. We know that after HIV infection, it takes many years to reach the stage of AIDS. There are no symptoms for a lengthy period of time.

There are some similarities and differences in genetic structure between HIV-1 and HIV-2. This difference is also seen in the disease progression. It is estimated that the genetic similarity between HIV-1 and HIV-2 ranges from 10% to 60%. The spikes of HIV1 are gp120 and gp41 molecules, while the spikes of HIV2 are gp105 and gp36 molecules. HIV1 has the p24 protein, while HIV2 has the p26 protein. 24 and 26 represent their molecular weights. There is a difference between HIV-1 and HIV-2. HIV-1 is transmitted from person to person about 10 times more effectively than HIV-2. HIV2 is relatively rare to transmit from mother to child when compared to HIV1.

There is a significant difference in the progression of the disease. HIV-1 devastates a person's immune system in 6 to 12 years. Whereas HIV-2 takes 10 to 20 years to shatter the immune system, this means that people who are infected with HIV-1 are likely to develop the disease much earlier. However, both types can eventually lead to AIDS.

Since HIV-2 is milder and progresses much more slowly than HIV-1, scientists had hoped for some time to develop a vaccine based on HIV-2. However, it was later evident that this was not feasible.

The C and E clades are most prevalent in India and South Asia, while the A and D clades are most prevalent in Africa. All these factors need to be considered in the development of drugs and vaccines.

All currently available antiretroviral drugs for HIV are active against HIV-1. However, some of these drugs are not effective against HIV-2. HIV-1 is an almost exclusive concern in industrialized countries, and the research is focused on developing medicines for HIV-1. A person infected with HIV-1 can also be infected with HIV-2. Conversely, an individual with HIV-2 can also contract HIV-1. It is important to recognize that an infected person may also be infected with another clade of the virus that gave rise to CRFs.

Diagnostic testing, as well as vaccine development, has become extraordinarily difficult due to the extreme genetic diversity in HIV. New recombinant strains may differ in fitness, transmissibility, and disease severity, and these differences need to be considered in the design of vaccine and drugs.

Chemokine Receptors: Gateways for HIV Entry

The establishment of HIV infection requires chemokine receptors (co-receptors) along with the CD4+ receptor. While one of these coreceptors, CCR5, is involved mainly in the transmission of HIV through sex, CXCR4 plays major role in transmission among injecting drug users.

4. Global impact of AIDS

AIDS is among the worst pandemics in recorded human history.

In the early days of AIDS, people believed the problem was insignificant because gay people and injecting drug users lived in small groups and made up a small minority. It was also believed that AIDS would not be a problem in developing and poor countries where homosexuality and injecting drug use were not widespread. Over time, other important catalysts for the spread of HIV, the virus that causes AIDS, have been identified. It was shown to be widespread, with signs of poverty such as illiteracy, ignorance, discrimination against women, malnutrition, and various social evils. Lack of awareness and lack of healthcare infrastructure such as diagnostic tests, preventive measures, counselling, and medical facilities are the main factors fuelling the spread of the disease.

Disparities Between Developed and Developing Nations:

Over the past four decades, the HIV/AIDS epidemic has evolved into a complex global challenge. There are significant disparities between developed and developing countries. Advancements in treatment and prevention have made it possible to control the spread of HIV in developed nations. Despite increased awareness, the epidemic continues to disproportionately impact resource-limited settings.

In developed countries, access to antiretroviral therapy and comprehensive prevention programs has significantly reduced HIV transmission rates and improved the quality of life for people living with HIV/AIDS. However, it is crucial to avoid the misconception that HIV is confined to specific groups or that it is no longer a significant concern. HIV affects individuals from all social classes, and ongoing efforts are needed to address health disparities and ensure equitable access to care and support for all affected communities.

Addressing the global HIV/AIDS epidemic requires a multifaceted approach that recognizes the unique challenges faced by different regions and populations. In developed countries, efforts should focus on ensuring equitable access to prevention and treatment services, combating stigma and discrimination, and addressing the needs of marginalized communities. For developing countries, strengthening healthcare systems, expanding access to affordable antiretroviral therapy, and promoting comprehensive prevention programs are crucial.

In contrast, developing countries, particularly those in sub-Saharan Africa, continue to bear the brunt of the epidemic. Factors such as poverty, limited healthcare infrastructure, social stigma, and gender inequality contribute to the high prevalence of HIV in these regions. The impact of AIDS on the working-age population has devastating consequences for economic development and social stability. Furthermore, the disease's effect on rural communities, often heavily reliant on agriculture, exacerbates challenges related to food security and poverty.

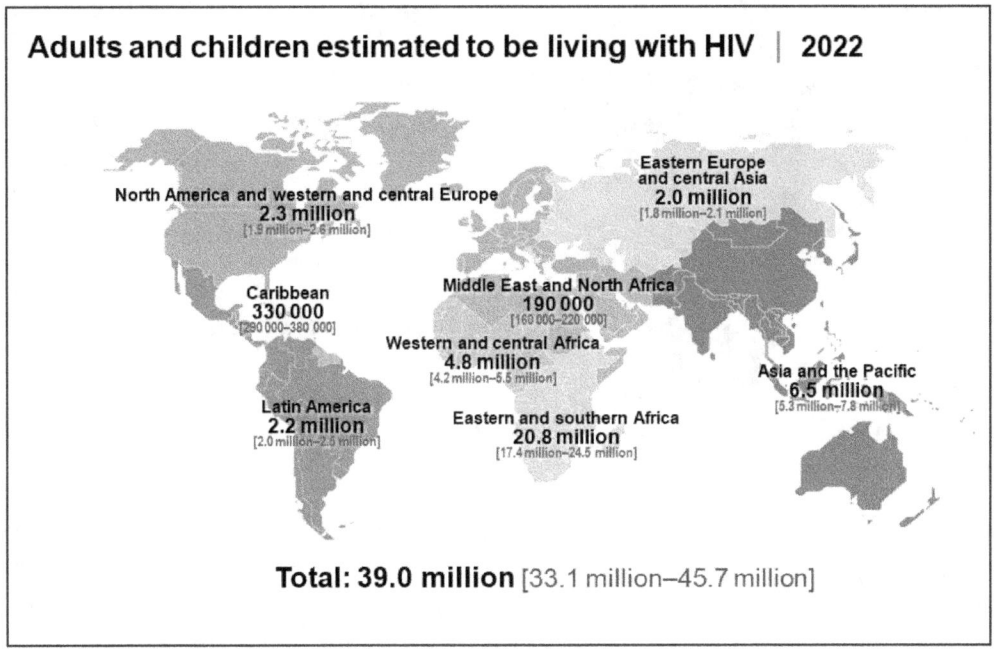

Ultimately, tackling the HIV/AIDS epidemic demands global solidarity and a commitment to human rights. By working together to address the underlying social and economic determinants of health, promoting education and awareness, and ensuring equitable access to prevention and treatment, we can strive towards a future where HIV/AIDS is no longer a threat to global health and well-being.

The Devastating Impact on African Countries: Between seven and 26 percent of adults in some African countries have HIV infection. All ten countries with the highest adult HIV prevalence in the world are African countries:

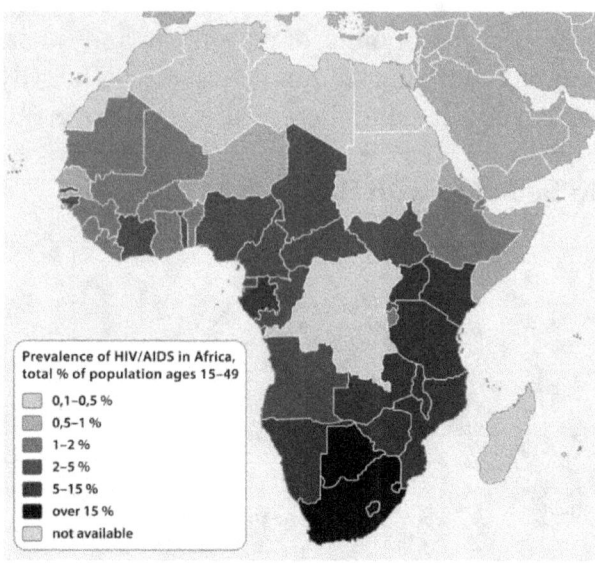

1. **Eswatini (formerly Swaziland) has the highest prevalence of HIV among adults, at 26 percent (25.9 percent). It is followed by 2. Lesotho (19.3%); 3. South Africa (17.8%); 4. Botswana (16.4%); 5. Mozambique (11.6%); 6. Zimbabwe (11%); 7. Namibia (11%); 8. Zambia (10.8%); 9. Malawi (7.1%) and 10. Equatorial Guinea (6.7%).**

The most tragic and deplorable conditions are in the societies of these African countries south of the Sahara Desert. Within a few years, all the progress that had been achieved for decades was wiped out by AIDS.

The loss of the working generation, i.e., workers and employees, due to AIDS and the inability to attend work due to the debility, had led to a production halt in some factories and offices. These countries are already economically weak. Some countries have witnessed financial collapse. The women and children of AIDS victims families were left in dire straits. In certain countries plagued by severe poverty, civil wars, and famines, AIDS has created a deplorable environment. The working class has diminished, leaving the elderly and children in a vulnerable position. They do not have enough resources to sustain their lives.

The grief of the families who lost their loved ones is unimaginable. Hundreds of thousands of babies were born with HIV infection. Such children do not have proper growth from the beginning and often fall ill and may die within a few years. In the early years of the epidemic, in African countries, family members of those who died from the disease were unable to perform their last rites and relied on charities and the government. This tragedy did not happen in a few days or months. For fifteen-twenty years, HIV, which spread like water undercurrent among the people of those African countries without their knowledge, surfaced as AIDS and created such a devastating and miserable situation. Had the United States not detected AIDS in 1981, the disease would have unleashed unimaginable devastation in African countries. Of the top 10 countries with the highest HIV/AIDS prevalence in the world, eight are in Africa.

Success Stories in HIV Prevention:

Uganda was the first country in the world to recognize the graveness of the AIDS epidemic, including the president and political figures. The AIDS Support Organization (TASO Uganda), founded in 1987, has been able to reduce the spread of HIV to a great extent with new approaches to combating the disease with patients actively involving themselves. After recognizing the sexual transmission of HIV in 1981, the use of condoms should have been promoted among sex workers in African countries, where HIV/AIDS has devastated economies and societies, which could have mitigated the tragedy.

For the first time in South Asia, Thailand's Prime Minister from 1991–92, Anand Panyarachun, along with the health minister, mandated the country's radio and TV broadcasts about AIDS prevention for half a minute every day. Condoms were made accessible to commercial sex workers as well as men. This has reduced the spread of HIV among sex workers by 90 percent in a short time. The Buddhist temple in Bangkok wrapped the ashes of AIDS patients in cloth and displayed them prominently. As a result, public awareness about AIDS has increased.

The Consequences of HIV Denialism:

Thabo Mbeki was president of South Africa from 1999 to 2008, during the height of the AIDS epidemic in sub-Saharan Africa. Peter Duesberg, a biology professor at the University of California, influenced him by promoting the idea that HIV was not the cause of AIDS. Mbeki asserted that poverty and malnutrition, not HIV, cause AIDS and mandated that people should not use the antiretroviral drugs prescribed for HIV. In addition, the government has stopped all government assistance to hospitals that provide HIV drugs to patients. The then health minister, Manto Tshabalala, advocated the use of alcohol, fruit, and vegetable decoctions as a treatment for AIDS. With the President himself saying that HIV is not the cause of AIDS, people ignored the risk of HIV infection with unsafe sex. HIV has spread throughout the country like wildfire. This tendency to deny facts has left South Africa with irreparable loss and endless tragedy. Jacob Zuma, who came to power in 2009, made antiretroviral drugs accessible to HIV-infected pregnant women and the elderly. It is estimated that more than 300,000 people have died due to a lack of treatment for HIV, which was available free of cost through international agencies. Now, South Africa has one of the highest HIV prevalences in the world. In South Africa, with a population of 62 million, there are 7.8 million people living with HIV/AIDS at the end of 2022, or 127 patients per 1,000 people.

AIDS and Advancements in Medical Science:

The HIV/AIDS pandemic has been a driving force behind significant advancements in medical approaches, including the acceleration of drug repurposing. Drug repurposing involves the application of an existing drug, originally developed for one disease, to treat another condition. A prime example of this approach is Azidothymidine (AZT or Zidovudine). Initially synthesized in 1964 as a potential anti-cancer drug, Azidothymidine failed to demonstrate efficacy against cancer. However, researchers in the mid-1980s discovered that the compound could inhibit the activity of the reverse transcriptase enzyme, which is crucial for the replication of HIV. After successful clinical trials demonstrated its effectiveness in suppressing HIV replication, the U.S. Food and Drug Administration (FDA) approved Zidovudine in March 1987 as the first antiretroviral drug for the treatment of HIV/AIDS. This approval marked a turning point in the management of the disease, paving the way for the development of more effective antiretroviral therapies and combination treatments. The prevention of infectious diseases mainly involves vaccines that prevent the damage caused by pathogens by preparing the immune system. Currently, there is no vaccine to prevent HIV infection. Experts have, however, developed a method to prevent infection by administering some of the HIV treatment drugs to individuals who are at risk of contracting the virus. This is called pre-exposure prophylaxis. Although this method is used on limited occasions for some infectious diseases, it is widely used in HIV prevention.

Only after many years of thorough and extensive research are new medicines approved for the treatment of an illness. Given the seriousness and life-threatening nature of AIDS, the rapid approval of drugs proven effective against HIV allowed for their immediate availability to patients. Recently, during the COVID crisis, some medicines received early approval prior to undergoing extensive research.

Sustain Action Against HIV/AIDS:

Natural disasters, which are a great tragedy for humanity, can occur without human involvement, and their damage is often impossible to prevent. HIV/AIDS, however, is a serious health issue whose rapid spread can be slowed or prevented through appropriate measures. The transmission of HIV can be controlled with basic precautions and cost-effective approaches. That is why all sectors of society—individuals, organizations, and governments—must make concerted efforts to address the factors contributing to the spread of HIV and ensure access to prevention, testing, and treatment services.

5. Routes of HIV infection

HIV can only be transmitted through the body fluids of an infected person. HIV is not spread by insects and social life.

Initially, researchers believed that AIDS exclusively affected gay men. Later, it was discovered that the human immunodeficiency virus (HIV), which causes AIDS, can be transmitted to others through the body fluids and secretions of those infected. However, many factors can affect this infection. Exchange of body fluids can usually occur during sex and in those taking injection drugs. Using contaminated needles, syringes, and blade or knife razors can also transmit HIV. An infected person whose HIV status was not determined can transmit the virus to others. Mothers can also pass on the infection to their offspring.

The HIV virus has an 'envelope' structure on its surface that contains the gp120 molecule. This gp120 molecule binds to the CD4+ protein found on certain cells in the human body, allowing the virus to infect those cells. CD4+ proteins are present on several types of white blood cells and play crucial roles in the immune system's defence against diseases.

These CD4+-expressing cells include helper T lymphocytes, regulatory T cells, macrophages, monocytes, and dendritic cells. Additionally, CD4+ proteins are present on specialized cells in various organs, such as Langerhans cells in the skin, Kupffer cells in the liver, microglia in the brain, and dendritic cells in Peyer's patches of the intestine.

Individuals who have recently contracted HIV infection are more likely to transmit the virus to others compared to those who have been living with HIV for a longer period of time. This increased transmissibility during the acute phase of infection is due to the higher viral loads present in the body before the immune system can mount an effective response.

Haemophilia patients are exposed to HIV by giving them factor VIII Concentrate from HIV-contaminated blood. In the United States, about half of all haemophiliacs, or 250,000 people, are infected with HIV.

Routes of HIV Transmission

Sexual Transmission:

- Genital Health and HIV Vulnerability
- Gender Disparities in Transmission Rates
- Impact of Other STIs and Genital Lesions
- Viral Load and Transmission Risk

The virus is present in high concentrations not only in the blood of HIV-infected people but also in semen and female genital secretions. In sexual intercourse, small, invisible cracks are formed in the genitals of the partners. Through these micro-ulcers, the virus spreads from one person to another.

The risk of infection is higher if either or both partners have a sexually transmitted disease. The reason for this is that the exchange of secretions from the ulcer occurs easily. In addition, the secretions contain CD4+ lymphocytes containing HIV. The risk of transmitting HIV through sex to healthy people from someone who does not have any diseases other than HIV infection is about 0.1 percent for a sexual encounter, which is a once in a thousand chance. However, this might not be the same case in rich and poor countries. Genital health is not good for most people in poor and developing countries. Genital diseases such as candidiasis and trichomoniasis are common among the people of these countries.

In women, a larger volume semen of the male reaches and remains for a longer time. So, if a man is infected with HIV, they can easily spread it to women through sex.

Several factors can affect HIV infection. The mucous membrane of the genital tract contains multiple layers of cells. Depending on the intensity of sexual activity, small tears or abrasions may form between the layers of mucosal cells, exposing the underlying lymphocytes and macrophages that contain CD4+ protein molecules. Additionally, Langerhans cells, which are a type of dendritic cells, are present in the mucosal layers.

The virus is present in high concentrations not only in the blood of HIV-infected people but also in semen and vaginal secretions. Through the semen or female genital secretions of an HIV-infected person, the virus penetrates through cracks in the genital mucosa of the sexual partner and attaches to CD4+ molecules. Depending on the level of readiness and force in the sexual act of the partners, there is a possibility of cracks forming in the genital membranes, which can lead to HIV infection.

A female sexual partner is ten times more likely to get HIV than a male sexual partner. Whether a person has an ulcer, an injury, or an infection, a large number of immune cells in the body reach that area to repair it. This is called inflammation. The debris of white blood cells damaged by the germs is seen as pus. If the person infected with HIV has an active disease, then the secretions and pus are copious, and the person can easily spread HIV.

If there are benign diseases, the lesions are rich in lymphocytes, macrophages, and Langerhans or Langerhans cells that contain the CD4+ molecule and can rapidly recruit HIV germs. This is because the rash appears more quickly and gives way to the virus. In cases where there is no sexual stimulation, there are more chances of injuries due to the lack of easy mating, and thus the probability of infection is also high.

However, if both sexual partners are not infected with HIV, there is no possibility of emergence HIV in them. The risk of HIV infection varies depending on the stage of infection. The reason for this depends on the concentration of the virus in the genital secretions and the concentration of HIV (viral load) in the patient's blood. The viral load in the blood depends on the stage of the disease. A high level of HIV in the blood and body fluids increases the risk of HIV infection. More than 90 percent of HIV infections in poor and developing countries are transmitted through heterosexual unprotected sex between infected men and women.

Having sex with an HIV-infected person during the first ten days of a woman's menstrual cycle increases the likelihood of contracting HIV for both partners. For the woman, the inner walls of the uterus are coarse and tender during this time, making transmission more likely. Similarly, an HIV-infected woman's menstrual blood poses a higher risk to her male partner.

During the first few weeks of HIV infection, the virus replicates exponentially. The body does not recognize the infection immediately, and the process of containing it has not yet begun. As a result, antibodies are not formed, and the virus replicates exponentially. Antibody tests are usually negative at this early stage. During this period, the virus is easily transmitted through sexual contact due to the high viral load.

Once the body's immune system detects the infection and produces antibodies, it partially restricts the replication of the virus. However, the virus is not eliminated entirely, and the person remains infected for life. In the advanced stage of HIV, known as AIDS, the viral load again reaches a high level. At this stage, the person can readily transmit HIV to others.

Although the chances of infecting others vary depending on the stage of the disease, once a person is infected with the virus, they can transmit it to others throughout their life. Despite the difference in transmission risk based on the disease progression, the infected individual remains a potential source of transmission indefinitely.

HIV primarily infects activated CD4++ T lymphocytes, which are a type of white blood cell crucial for immune function. In healthy individuals, only about 1% to 5% of these cells are in an activated state. However, during illnesses caused by infectious diseases, a higher proportion (up to 20%) of CD4++ T cells becomes activated. Consequently, if an individual has sexual contact with an HIV-infected person while suffering from another infection, the probability of acquiring HIV increases.

HIV transmission is more efficient among men who have sex with men (MSM). This is due to a higher likelihood of minor injuries and abrasions in the mucosal membranes during anal intercourse, which can facilitate viral entry. Sexual contact between men is one of the primary modes of HIV transmission in Western societies.

Mother-to-Child Transmission (MTCT):
- Pregnancy, Delivery, and Breastfeeding Risks
- Prevention Strategies for MTCT

A woman living with HIV can potentially transmit the virus to her baby during pregnancy, delivery of baby, or breastfeeding. The risk of mother-to-child transmission ranges from 11% to 35%, depending on factors such as access to antiretroviral treatment and appropriate medical care. However, with effective preventive measures, the transmission risk can be significantly reduced. Currently, mother-to-child transmission is a significant mode of HIV spread in some regions.

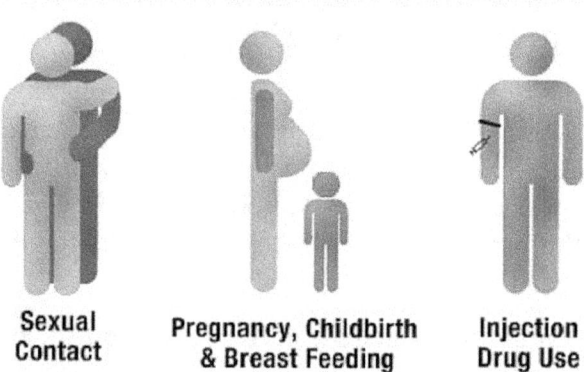

Transmission Through Contaminated Needles and Sharps:
- Injection Drug Use and Needle Sharing
- Healthcare Settings and Occupational Exposure

HIV can be transmitted to uninfected individuals through the use of contaminated needles, syringes, or other sharp instruments that have been exposed to the blood or bodily fluids of a person living with HIV. Improper sterilization and handling of medical equipment can pose a risk. Healthcare workers can also be at risk of occupational exposure if proper safety protocols are not followed when handling sharps or bodily fluids.

Sharing needles or other injection equipment among people who inject drugs can facilitate HIV transmission if one person is infected. This mode of transmission has contributed significantly to HIV spread in various eastern-Europe countries and northeast region of India.

It is important to note that with proper precautions, such as access to sterile injection equipment, the risk of transmission can be minimized.

Other Potential Routes of Transmission:

- Blood Transfusions and Organ Transplants
- Tattooing and Body Piercing
- Debunking Myths: Casual Contact and Insect Bites

In healthcare settings, HIV can be transmitted through unscreened blood transfusions or the use of contaminated needles or other medical equipment. Proper screening and sterilization protocols are crucial to prevent such occurrences.

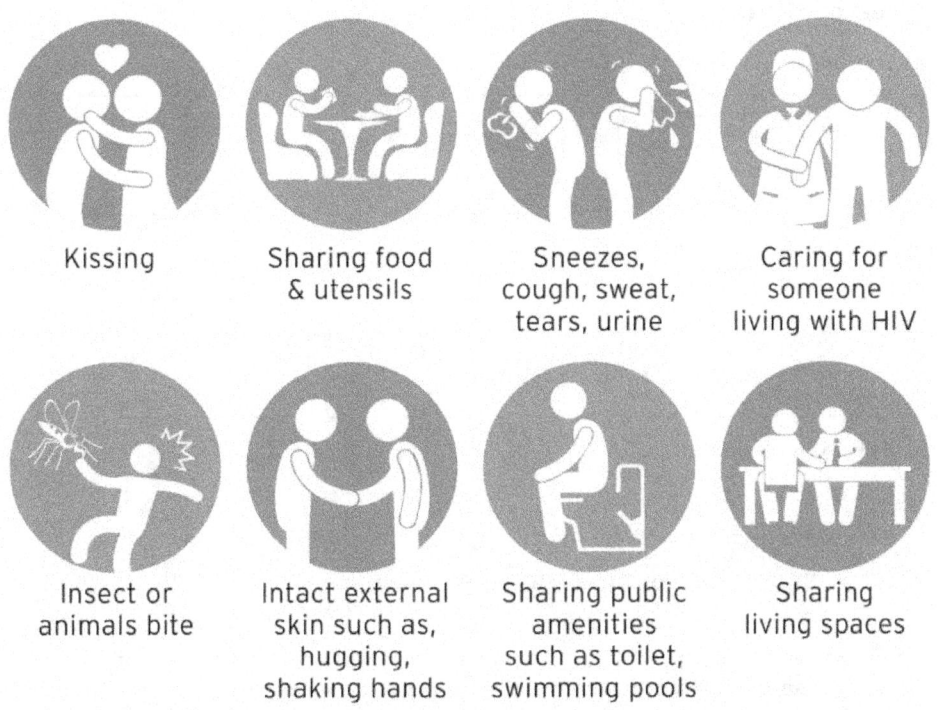

There is also a risk of HIV transmission during procedures involving needles, such as tattooing or body piercing, if contaminated equipment is used.

It is important to note that HIV is not spread through casual contact, water, air, or insect bites. The virus is only transmitted when specific bodily fluids (blood, semen, vaginal fluids, or breast milk) from an infected person enter the bloodstream of another individual.

The primary modes of HIV transmission are sexual contact (heterosexual or homosexual) and mother-to-child transmission during pregnancy, delivery, or breastfeeding. Sharing of contaminated needles or injection equipment among people who inject drugs is another significant mode of transmission.

Statistical Overview of Transmission Risks:

The Centers for Disease Control, US estimate that the probability of becoming infected with HIV per 10,000 people who participate in activities that could potentially infect:

Transmission Route	Possible infections 10,000 exposures
Sharing of needles during injection drug use	63
By Needlestick injury from an HIV-positive patient	23
To Passive partner in male gay sex	138
To active partner in male gay sex	11
To Woman having sex with an HIV-infected man	8
To man having sex with an HIV-infected woman	4
HIV transmission through blood transfusion (estimated cases)	9,250

Chances of HIV infection in oral sex is negligible (lower risk).

It is crucial to understand that any exposure carries a risk, and preventive measures should always be taken. While the chances of transmission may seem low in some cases, the consequences can be severe. Therefore, it is essential to practice safe behaviours and seek appropriate medical care and support services to minimize the risk of HIV transmission.

6. HIV Prevention Methods

Simple and accessible methods can effectively prevent HIV/AIDS.

The Importance of Prevention:
- Understanding HIV Transmission Routes
- The Role of Asymptomatic Carriers
- Taking Precautions: A Shared Responsibility

HIV infection occurs when the bodily fluids (blood, semen, vaginal fluids, or breast milk) of an infected person enter another individual. One cannot determine an individual's HIV infection solely by their appearance. Infected individuals can remain without health issues (asymptomatic) for many years. However, approximately 12 percent of individuals with HIV are undiagnosed at any given time. Despite being unaware of their status, they can still transmit the virus to others through their bodily fluids. Therefore, in any situation where an exchange of bodily fluids is possible, suitable precautions should be taken to prevent such an exchange.

Preventing Sexual Transmission:
- Abstinence and Monogamy
- Condom Use: Male and Female Options
- Male Circumcision: Reducing Acquisition Risk
- Microbicidal Gels: Emerging Technologies

Currently, more than 90 percent of HIV infections are transmitted through sexual contact with an infected person. To prevent this, it is advisable to practice abstinence or mutual monogamy with an uninfected partner. In non-monogamous sexual relationships, the proper and consistent use of a new condom for each sexual act can effectively prevent the exchange of genital fluids and secretions, greatly reducing the risk of HIV transmission. Using condoms in such situations should be viewed as a responsible act of self-care and caring for others, rather than a lack of trust. When used correctly, condoms provide over 90% protection against HIV and other sexually transmitted infections (STIs), including Hepatitis B and C. Condoms can also serve as an effective contraceptive method.

There are two types of condoms: male condoms and female condoms. Male condoms (also called external condoms) are more commonly used. Female condoms (also known as internal condoms) offer an alternative option for women, particularly in situations where negotiating condom use with a partner or client is difficult.

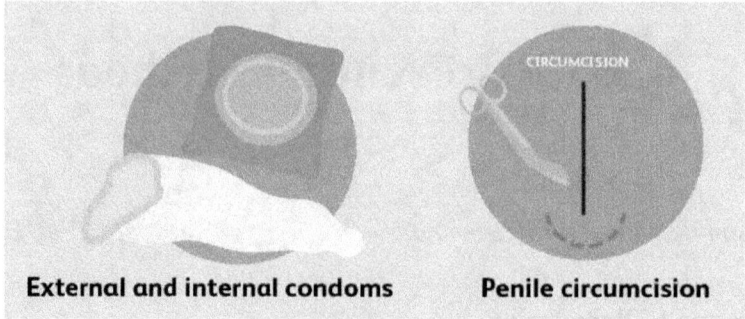

External and internal condoms **Penile circumcision**

Male circumcision has been shown to reduce the risk of HIV acquisition by approximately 50% due to the removal of the foreskin, which has a high concentration of Langerhans or Langerhans cells (which contain CD4+ receptors necessary for HIV entry). In some African countries, this traditional practice has contributed to decreasing HIV transmission rates.

Research is ongoing to develop effective microbicidal gels that can further reduce the risk of HIV infection, particularly for individuals engaged in sex work.

Preventing Mother-to-Child Transmission (MTCT):

- Family Planning and Pregnancy Prevention
- Antiretroviral Treatment for Pregnant Women
- Safe Infant Feeding Practices

Another mode of HIV transmission is from an infected mother to her child during pregnancy, labour, or breastfeeding. HIV-positive women can prevent this by avoiding pregnancy or, if desired, seeking appropriate medical guidance and treatment to minimize the risk of transmission. In cases of unwanted pregnancy, abortion may be considered. HIV-positive mothers are advised to formula-feed their infants, as breastfeeding carries a risk of transmission. However, in resource-limited settings where access to clean water is scarce, formula feeding may increase the risk of other infectious diseases, leading to higher infant mortality rates. In such cases, breastfeeding may be the safer option, as the risk of HIV transmission through breastmilk is relatively low.

Preventing Transmission Through Contaminated Needles:

- Sterile Injection Equipment in Healthcare
- Harm Reduction Strategies for Drug Users
- Safe Practices for Professionals Using Sharps

In healthcare settings, the use of sterile, disposable needles and syringes is crucial to preventing HIV transmission. If reusing equipment is unavoidable, proper sterilization through boiling or chemical disinfection is necessary. Barbers and other professionals who use sharp instruments should follow similar sterilization protocols between clients.

Regarding blood transfusions, it is advisable to receive blood from trusted relatives or friends who practice safe behaviours after proper screening for HIV and other infectious agents. In emergency situations where a designated donor is unavailable, blood from licensed blood banks can be used after appropriate testing.

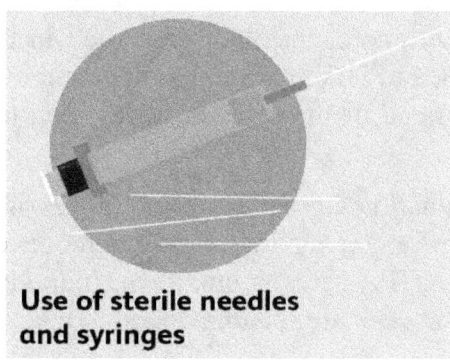

Use of sterile needles and syringes

By following these preventive measures and promoting awareness, the spread of HIV/AIDS can be effectively controlled.

Safe Blood Transfusions and Organ Transplants:

During medical operations or accidents involving severe bleeding, patients may require blood transfusions. In such cases, it is advisable to receive blood from blood banks where it is screened for various diseases. However, even this screening process is not 100% safe.

It takes 6 to 12 weeks for a person infected with HIV to develop detectable antibodies against the virus. This period is known as the "window period." During this window period, which typically lasts 3 to 6 weeks but can extend longer, standard antibody tests cannot accurately diagnose HIV infection. This creates a critical gap in detection, as individuals can unknowingly transmit the virus to others while testing negative for HIV antibodies.

Currently, in the blood banks of developing and poor countries, including India, only antibody tests are performed. These tests cannot detect HIV during the window period before antibodies develop. Even if the blood tests negative for HIV antibodies, the recipient can still become infected with HIV if the donated blood is from someone in the window period.

Therefore, it cannot be said that the tests conducted in blood banks are 100% safe for detecting HIV. In developed countries, blood banks use antigen tests, which can detect HIV earlier than antibody tests, before the window period ends. This makes the blood supply safer in developed countries.

The use of contaminated needles during tattooing can transmit HIV. However, now it is a good development to use disposable needles in many instances.

Emerging Prevention Strategies:
- Pre-Exposure Prophylaxis (PrEP)
- Post-Exposure Prophylaxis (PEP)
- Treatment as Prevention (TasP) and U=U

Since 2011, innovative approaches have emerged in HIV prevention. People who are potentially exposed to HIV infection are given preventive treatment with a two-drug combination instead of the three-drug regimen that is usually given for regular HIV treatment.

This two-drug combination of antiretroviral drugs is used as pre-exposure prophylaxis (PrEP) before engaging in sexual intercourse with an HIV-positive partner or a person whose HIV status is unknown. Individuals who have a risk of exposure more than once a week are recommended to take PrEP regularly.

When one partner has HIV infection and the other is HIV negative (a discordant couple or mixed status couple), HIV drugs are given to the infected person regardless of their CD4+ lymphocyte count to reduce the likelihood of HIV transmission. Even if the HIV-positive partners occasionally do not follow protective practices, their negative partners are less likely to acquire HIV due to the undetectable viral load. This is called 'treatment as prevention' or 'U=U' (Undetectable = Untransmissible).

After a potential HIV exposure incident, doctors administer a combination of two drugs for four weeks to prevent infection. This is called post-exposure prophylaxis (PEP). After sexual contact with a person of unknown HIV status, or if a condom breaks during intercourse, PEP can protect against contracting HIV.

Currently, the 'Treatment as Prevention' protocol is being widely adopted to prevent HIV transmission. Studies have shown that reducing the viral load in an HIV-positive patient to undetectable levels virtually eliminates the risk of HIV transmission to their partner. In developed countries, where HIV primarily affects certain groups, this approach has shown great results.

The Role of Antiretroviral Drugs in Prevention:

Pre-exposure prophylaxis (PrEP) involves two types that address different needs. On-demand PrEP involves the administration of antiretrovirals both before and after potential exposure to HIV infection. Those at risk are given a '2-1-1' regimen: one tablet 24 hours before the potential exposure to sexual activity or injection drug use, one more tablet two hours before the event, one pill immediately after the risk event, and another pill within 24 hours after the event. The other PrEP is for those who encounter such potential events more than once a week and receive a combination of two drugs for regular use. Recently, the FDA approved the single-drug Cabotegravir injection for use as pre-exposure prophylaxis once every two months.

Tenofovir and Emtricitabine tablets are a common combination in both 'pre-exposure prophylaxis' (PrEP) and 'post-exposure prophylaxis' (PEP). These drugs inhibit the reverse transcriptase enzyme, which is crucial for the conversion of viral RNA to DNA during the HIV replication cycle. By preventing this step, they halt viral replication before the integration of the viral genome into the host cell's DNA and before HIV can become a part of the human genome. Once HIV has integrated into the human DNA, it is impossible to eliminate the infection. This is why protease inhibitors, which are effective against new virions produced after integration into the host DNA, are not useful in PrEP and PEP. Cabotegravir injection is also a drug that works by preventing the integration of the viral DNA into the human DNA. Studies have shown that pre-exposure prophylaxis reduces the risk of HIV infection by about 80%.

Overcoming Stigma and Promoting Awareness:

- Respecting the Rights of HIV/AIDS Patients
- Early Testing and Treatment
- Community Support and Education Initiatives

It is everyone's responsibility to fully control the spread of HIV by following appropriate HIV prevention strategies, such as consistent and correct condom use, access to PrEP and PEP when necessary, and regular testing for early detection and treatment.

Controlling the spread of HIV is a shared responsibility that requires a comprehensive approach to prevention strategies. Consistent and correct condom use, access to pre-exposure prophylaxis (PrEP) and post-exposure prophylaxis (PEP) when needed, and regular HIV testing for early detection and prompt treatment are crucial measures that everyone should prioritize.

Stigmatization of individuals living with HIV/AIDS is a significant barrier that can contribute to the further spread of the virus. When communities embrace a non-judgmental and supportive attitude towards HIV patients, respecting their rights and dignity, it facilitates timely access to medical care and effective control of the epidemic. Uganda, despite its limited resources, has demonstrated the positive impact of such an approach on curbing HIV transmission.

The fear of social rejection and discrimination can discourage individuals from seeking healthcare services, leading to a delay in diagnosis and treatment. Undiagnosed or untreated HIV infections increase the risk of transmission to others, especially during the later stages when viral loads are higher. Therefore, it is essential to challenge and eliminate the stigma surrounding HIV/AIDS, creating an environment where individuals feel safe and encouraged to seek testing, treatment, and support without fear of discrimination.

By fostering a compassionate and inclusive society, we can break down barriers, ensure timely access to essential prevention and treatment measures, and collectively work towards controlling the spread of HIV while upholding the rights and dignity of those affected. Early diagnosis help prevent further spread.

7. The ravage of AIDS

The devastation and destruction that HIV caused is unimaginable and can only be prevented with awareness and accessible policies.

The Global Burden of HIV/AIDS:

Statistics on HIV / AIDS are compiled and published every two years by UNAIDS - the United Nations Joint Program on AIDS.

UNAIDS report estimates by the end of 2022:

85.5 million people worldwide were infected with HIV.

More than 40.4 million people had lost their lives to AIDS.

About 15 million of them were children under the age of 14.

In 2022, 1.3 million people were newly diagnosed with HIV. 630,000 people died of AIDS.

Two million people died of AIDS in 2004. Globally, 53 percent of people living with HIV were women and girls.

The highest number of people diagnosed with AIDS in its 43-year history was 3.2 million in 1995. As a result of concerted global efforts to prevent the spread of HIV, new infections have since declined by nearly 59%.

Globally, 29.8 million people, or 76% of those infected, receiving antiretroviral therapy. 9.2 million people still do not have access to HIV drugs. About 77 percent of adults who are diagnosed with HIV take medications. Only 57 out of 100 children under the age of 14 receive HIV medications. The reason for this situation is the lack of adequate availability of paediatric formulations

Out of 100 individuals infected with HIV, only 88 have been diagnosed. The remaining individuals remain undiagnosed. Globally, 0.7 percent of people over the age of 14 are living with HIV.

High percentage people in certain Risk groups are affected:
- 2.5% of commercial sex workers
- 7.5% of gay people
- 5% injectable drug users
- 10.3% of transgender people
- 1.4% of imprisoned.

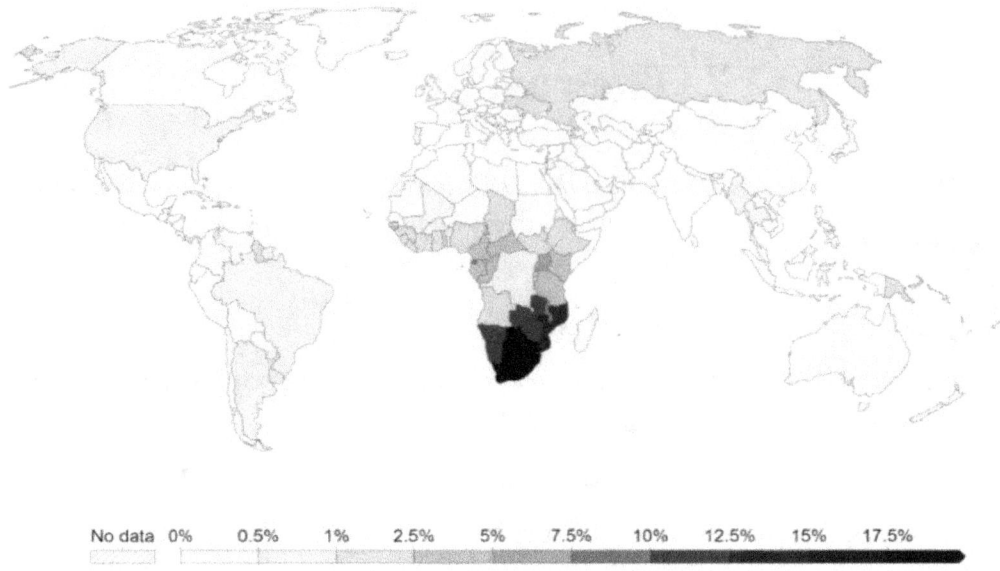

HIV prevalence in the world (more prevalent in countries shown in darker colour.

The Impact on Different Regions:

• Africa: The Epicentre of the Epidemic

Countries with the Highest HIV Prevalence:

1. **South Africa:** 7.6 million people
2. **India:** 2.5 million people
3. **Mozambique:** 2.4 million people
4. **Nigeria:** 2.07 million people
5. **Tanzania:** 1.7 million people
6. **Zambia:** 1.4 million people
7. **Uganda:** 1.4 million people
8. **Kenya:** 1.4 million people
9. **Zimbabwe:** 1.3 million people
10. **USA:** 1.07 million people
11. **Malawi:** 1 million people

About a quarter (23%) of new HIV infections occur among people aged 15 to 25. Every day, about 3,500 people worldwide contract HIV, which equates to about 145 new infections every hour. 90% of them are from developing and poor countries.

Africa is home to 18% of the world's population. However, two-thirds of new HIV infections occur in African countries. In countries with a high prevalence of AIDS, more than two-thirds of deaths between the ages of 20 and 45 are due to AIDS.

The Human Cost of HIV/AIDS:

Economic Hardship and Loss of Livelihood

Social Stigma and Discrimination

Psychological Impact on Individuals & Families

Infectious diseases are primarily acute. Most of these diseases last a few days to weeks. However, treatment for tuberculosis can take six to twelve months to completely cure the infection. Hepatitis B and hepatitis C, which were once considered chronic diseases, are now curable. Many global crises create havoc for a limited period. However, HIV is a chronic, lifelong disease. As a result, HIV-infected individuals and their families face economic hardship due to the need for continued treatment and occasional illnesses associated with the infection. Without access to timely and effective treatment, HIV can lead to serious complications and ultimately prove fatal.

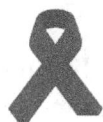

Dr. Yanamadala Murali Krishna

8. AIDS: The Indian scenario

With the presence of all catalysing factors, the disease spread rapidly in India.

An underestimated menace:

- India's HIV/AIDS Burden: Second Highest Globally
- The Role of Poverty, Inequality, and Social Stigma

While Africa continues to be devastated, AIDS is spreading in South Asia and Eastern Europe. Apart from the prevalence of extramarital sex, which contributes to the spread of HIV in India, there are certain special circumstances that contribute to the spread of AIDS. In India, numerous factors contribute to the spread of AIDS, including poverty, lack of HIV awareness, gender discrimination, illiteracy, inadequate sexual health education, malnutrition, and social taboos surrounding discussions about sex. All these adverse conditions act as catalysts, facilitating the rapid transmission of HIV within Indian communities.

Poverty is a major driving force behind the HIV epidemic in the country, as it limits access to healthcare, education, and resources for prevention and treatment. The lack of equitable access to health services for all people and inadequate access to HIV prevention strategies and resources for vulnerable populations also contribute to the spread of the virus. Some youths in our country's northeastern states engage in injecting drug use. Despite their smaller numbers, they frequently share needles and syringes. Therefore, once the virus enters these groups, it spreads rapidly among them. If some of these youths engage in sex work or come into contact with sex workers, the risk of HIV transmission increases significantly. Sex workers are at a higher risk of contracting and transmitting HIV, which can contribute to the spread of the virus in the wider community.

Catalysts for Transmission:

- Lack of Awareness and Education
- Gender Discrimination and Harmful Practices
- Injection Drug Use and Needle Sharing
- Sex Work and Vulnerable Populations

HIV infection in India was first diagnosed among sex workers in Chennai in 1986. Despite the late identification of the disease, by the end of 2022, India has the second-highest number of infected people in the world. There are 2.5 million people living with HIV/AIDS in India. Organized prostitution is illegal in India. However, some girls and women are forced into this profession. In such contexts, they cannot compel their clients to use condoms to protect themselves from HIV and other sexually transmitted infections. In some parts of our country, there were evil practices like Basivi, Jogini, and Devadasi. These inhuman practices, carried out in the name of God, compelled some women to become the joint property of society and serve men for their happiness. This is a form of sex work. Such malpractices also contribute to the spread of HIV.

The National AIDS Control Organization (NACO) has conducted tests among pregnant women across the country to assess the extent of the spread of HIV in a large country like India, which has the world's largest population and diverse traditions. Pregnancy in India is usually associated with family life. Usually, women acquire HIV through their husbands only. Knowing the HIV infection rate among pregnant women can provide a realistic estimate of the HIV prevalence in society. India has the second-highest number of HIV-infected people in the world after South Africa (7.6 million). The fact that the virus has already spread not only among sex workers and injecting drug users, who are considered high-risk groups, but also among the general population in our society, shows the seriousness of the problem.

In developing and poor countries, including India, HIV is most commonly transmitted through heterosexual sexual contact between men and women.

AIDS is tearing apart families. Millions of children are orphaned. We must tackle AIDS, a disease for which there is no cure and no vaccine in the near future, unitedly and effectively. Experiences not only from industrialized and wealthy countries but also from developing countries such as Uganda and Thailand show that the spread of HIV can be reduced by raising awareness of HIV among the masses. HIV patients in developed countries typically infected with rare opportunistic germs only when their immune system is severely damaged, because viral, bacterial, fungal, and parasitic diseases are rare among their general populace. As a result, in developed countries, people infected with the disease develop AIDS after 10 to 20 years. However, due to the high prevalence of various infections in developing and poor countries, HIV-infected individuals are more susceptible to infection when their immune system weakens. In poor countries, the disease progresses rapidly, reaching AIDS within 6 to 12 years.

HIV patients in these countries are highly vulnerable to tuberculosis, which is the biggest public health problem in poor and developing nations, including India. AIDS cases are on the rise in our country.

Regional Disparities and High-Risk Groups:

According to the National AIDS Control Organization, India HIV Estimates 2021, the adult (15–49 years) HIV prevalence rate in India is 0.21% nationally. However, some states have much higher prevalence, such as Mizoram (2.70%),

Nagaland (1.36%), Manipur (1.05%), Andhra Pradesh (0.67%), and Telangana (0.47%).

Adult HIV prevalence and People Living with HIV number by Estimates by State/UT2021

S No	State/ Union Territory	Percentage of adult HIV Prevalence (15-49 yrs.)	Total number of PLHIV (Highest estimate – Lowest estimate)
1	Andhra Pradesh	0.67 (0.56-0.79)	3,21,02(2,77,878-3,71,721)
2	Arunachal Pradesh	0.07 (0.04-0.10)	686 (453-1,001)
3	Assam	0.09 (0.08-0.11)	25,073 (22,137-28,765)
4	Bihar	0.16 (0.11-0.22)	1,42,793 (95,813-1,97,035)
5	Chhattisgarh	0.17 (0.14-0.22)	39,626(33,108-49,177)
6	Delhi	0.31 (0.25-0.39)	55,801 (45,529-68,592)
7	Goa	0.31 (0.24-0.41)	4,596 (3,838-5,657)
8	Gujarat	0.19 (0.16-0.23)	1,13,532 (93,717-1,38,484)
9	Himachal Pradesh	0.11 (0.08-0.13)	7,139 (5,575-8,649)
10	Haryana	0.22 (0.18-0.26)	49,976 (42,025-60,665)
11	Jharkhand	0.08 (0.06-0.11)	24,671 (17,439-32,999)
12	Jammu & Kashmir	0.06 (0.03-0.10)	65,28 (3,795-10,213)
13	Ladakh		
14	Karnataka	0.46 (0.40-0.56)	275,880(2,39,573-3,23,246)
15	Kerala	0.06 (0.04-0.09)	21,211 (15,360-28,030)
16	Meghalaya	0.42 (0.25-0.69)	8,692 (5,178-14,341)
17	Maharashtra	0.33 (0.28-0.39)	3,94,077(3,40,735-4,56,573)

HIV-AIDS

18	Manipur	1.05 (0.92-1.22)	27,989 (24,472-31,770)
19	Madhya Pradesh	0.08 (0.07-0.10)	54,773 (47,799-65,551)
20	Mizoram	2.70 (2.24-3.25)	23,802 (19,783-28,481)
21	Nagaland	1.36 (1.08-1.85)	21,730 (17,402-29,067)
22	Odisha	0.14 (0.10-0.19)	52,109 (38,709-68,535)
23	Punjab	0.28 (0.23-0.35)	72,954 (60,267-88,676)
24	Rajasthan	0.10 (0.09-0.12)	67,186 (56,181-79,842)
25	Sikkim	0.09 (0.05-0.14)	468 (271-767)
26	Tamil Nadu	0.22 (0.18-0.24)	1,62,857(1,37,575-1,80,868)
27	Tripura	0.12 (0.08-0.16)	3,608 (2,358-4,731)
28	Uttarakhand	0.12 (0.10-0.15)	11,327 (9,414-14,059)
29	Uttar Pradesh	0.10 (0.08-0.14)	178134(1,38,518-2,35,662)
30	West Bengal	0.08 (0.07-0.09)	69,199 (62,518-77,640)
31	A & N Islands	0.14 (0.06-0.38)	426 (195-1,153)
32	Chandigarh	0.19 (0.13-0.26)	1,921 (1,415-2,599)
33	DNH&DD	0.19 (0.13-0.25)	1,543 (1,076-2,087)
34	Puducherry	0.31 (0.18-0.46)	3,962 (2,459-5,761)
35	Telangana	0.47 (0.37-0.60)	1,55,991(1,29,316-1,94,132)
	India	**0.21 (0.17-0.25)**	**24,01,284(19,92,058-29,06,772)**

The spread of HIV is a massive economic burden for India. Every responsible citizen should consider AIDS prevention a social obligation and work tirelessly towards it. In every possible context, the media, along with those in the political, administrative, medical, and non-governmental sectors, must play an appropriate role in raising public awareness about AIDS. We should pass on the fruits of development to the next generation.

Due to inherent limitations, it is not possible to determine the exact number of people infected with HIV in the country. We follow certain methodologies to arrive at realistic estimates. Based on information from our National AIDS Control Organization and the June 1998 UNAIDS report, our country had 4.1 million HIV-positive individuals, the highest number in the world at that time.

According to the December 2022 UNAIDS report, there were an estimated 2.5 million people living with HIV in India. It is evident from the data that the estimates of the number of people living with HIV in India have fluctuated over the years, potentially due to various factors such as changes in methodologies, data collection, and the actual spread of the virus. By now, the system had perfected the methodology, and the present figure shows a realistic number. AIDS is a lifelong disease that primarily affects reproductive age groups, contributing to economic productivity and country development while necessitating more effective and vigorous prevention programmes.

9. HIV-AIDS

AIDS is a serious, life-threatening illness that occurs many years after a person is infected with HIV.

The Progression of HIV: Three-Stages of Disease

The immune system of HIV-infected people gradually weakens. There are many microorganisms present in the air, water, and atmosphere around us. These include bacteria, viruses, fungi, parasites, etc. Most of them are not harmful to us.

While some infections can cause illnesses ranging from trivial to fatal. When these germs enter a person, the cells of the immune system in that individual fight those germs and protect the person from falling ill. In the fight between pathogens and the immune system, several factors play a role. The health condition of the person, age, the number of germs entering the body, their strength, etc., are factors that contribute to the causation of the disease. In people infected with HIV, CD4+ lymphocytes and macrophages, which play a pivotal role in the immune system, are reduced, and some of them are defective and do not function properly. Therefore, in HIV patients, the immune system is often overwhelmed by the causative agent in many instances. Hence, HIV-infected people are easily susceptible to infections.

The natural history of HIV is the changes that it undergoes and the changes that it causes in a person's body after HIV infection.

Stage 1 (Acute HIV Infection):

Some people develop a flu-like illness within 1-2 weeks after being infected with HIV. Symptoms may include fever, sore throat, red rash on the body, hives, and swelling of the lymph nodes in the neck and groin areas. This is called Acute HIV infection. Many types of viruses and colds have identical symptoms. Therefore, it is difficult to predict whether a fever could be due to HIV. Only about 30 percent of people infected with HIV experience this acute illness. However, in this early stage, the virus replicates unchecked, and the HIV load in the patient's body reaches high levels. Large numbers of HIV-infected lymphocytes reach the lymph nodes. In most cases, patients and doctors consider it to be a mild viral infection, such as the flu or infectious mononucleosis. The HIV viral load increases tremendously in the first two months. The patient's immune system controls the viral replication to some extent within six months.

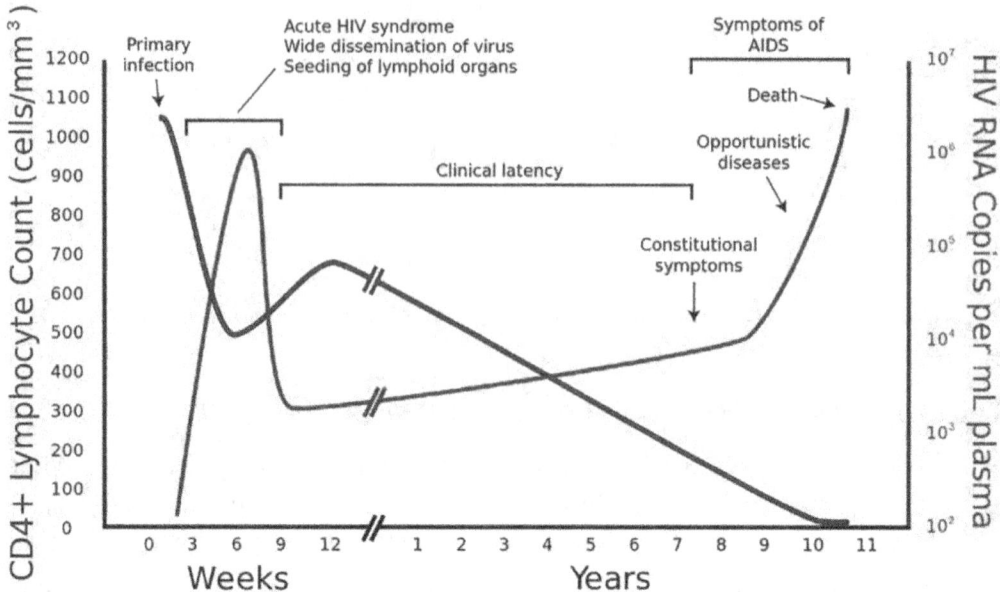

Stage 2 (Clinical Latency):

The second stage is called the latent period or clinical latency. In developed countries, it lasts 10 to 15 years after the first stage. In developing countries, the average latent period is 6-12 years. During this period, the virus multiplies exponentially. The growing virus gradually destroys CD4+ lymphocytes and other cells that bear the CD4+ protein. The falling number of CD4+ cells means decreasing immunity, making the patient susceptible to various diseases. In the stage when CD4+ lymphocyte counts are between 200 and 500 per microliter, there is not much difficulty for patients in developed countries. However, in countries where infections are prevalent, many pathogens often attack the person's body at this stage. The patient may suffer from different types of skin diseases, such as sores, abscesses, herpes zoster, molluscum contagiosum, warts, severe itching, extensive ringworm (tinea), and fungal infections of the nails. Although these are not life-threatening, they can create a sense of stigma towards these patients in the community, leading to depression. Oral candidiasis (white coating in the mouth) may occur. Patients may get repeatedly ill and experience swelling of the lymph nodes in the armpits, groin, and neck.

Some patients may suffer from serious diseases such as tuberculosis, pneumonia, and typhoid. If not treated on time, these can be life-threatening.

Stage 3 (AIDS): The third stage is the AIDS stage. According to the Centers for Disease Control and Prevention (CDC) in 1987, AIDS is defined as a condition in which HIV patients have less than 200 CD4+ lymphocytes per microliter, or less than 14% of total lymphocytes, and/or the presence of any designated severe infectious disease or cancer. However, it now seems inappropriate to define AIDS solely based on the number of CD4+ lymphocytes without severe illness. AIDS is a medical epidemiological term that needs to be limited to administrative contexts and used primarily by governments. A person infected with HIV will gradually lose weight. In the early years, a fever for more than a month, diarrhoea for more than a month, and weight loss of more than 10% within a month were considered indicators of AIDS.

Opportunistic Infections: Exploiting a Weakened Defence

These infectious diseases are usually prevalent in the community and environment around the patient. Microorganisms that cause infectious diseases are rare in the environments of rich countries such as the United States and Europe. According to the health standards of the people in those countries, it is also very rare for them to be afflicted with infectious diseases. Since bacterial, fungal, viral, and parasitic infections are relatively rare in developed countries, HIV patients in those countries can only become infected when their immunity is low enough that they get sick from weak germs present in the environment, which do not cause disease in healthy people. These are known as opportunistic infections. Additionally, HIV patients in developed countries are susceptible to certain types of rare cancers. Usually, when cancer cells start developing in a person, their immune system controls it. However, due to a weakened immune system, HIV patients are more susceptible to rare cancers. Opportunistic infections are rare diseases that occur only in conditions where immunity is almost non-existent. In the United States, a new immune-deficient disease (AIDS) was identified with the identification of clusters of the rare lung fungal infection *Pneumocystis carinii* (now *Pneumocystis jiroveci*) * and the rare Kaposi's sarcoma cancer**.

Global Divide: AIDS in Developed vs. Developing Nations

But in poor and developing countries, the situation is different. In the atmosphere of these countries, there are many different types of microorganisms at a very high level. Bacteria, viruses, fungi, and parasitic diseases are prevalent in these communities. Since any disease must be transmitted from the surrounding environment, HIV patients in poor developing countries are exposed to a large variety of infectious diseases and are at risk of acquiring them. In fact, although the germs that cause disease in HIV patients in industrialized countries are very weak, they only cause disease because the patients' immune systems are destroyed. That is why, in the pre-AIDS era, these diseases were seen only on very rare occasions. Research, awareness, and medicines related to them are very limited. The prices of medicines to treat those rare diseases are also very high. Even though there are no medicines for some diseases, the patient's body can get rid of the infection if the number of CD4+ lymphocytes improves.

After starting HIV medicines, even without specific treatment for some opportunistic infections, the body can fight off the disease. The most common diseases among HIV patients in developing and poor countries are the same diseases that occur in others in the communities there. Hence, suitable drugs are available for most of the diseases that occur in HIV patients of third-world countries. Additionally, HIV patients in these countries are exposed much earlier to tuberculosis, bacteria that cause pneumonia, and diarrhoea. Thus, it is possible to diagnose HIV much earlier. The severity of any disease is higher in HIV patients, and the disease progresses faster than in others. Only a very small percentage of those infected with HIV develop rare infectious diseases that occur in rich countries. Rare diseases that occur in rich countries are too expensive to diagnose and treat, so people here cannot afford them. It is like a small relief in big trouble.

The Spectrum of AIDS-Related Illnesses:

AIDS is not just a single disease. An HIV-infected individual may be afflicted with many diseases at different stages of falling immunity. Therefore, it cannot be said that AIDS is the same disease for all people. The same pathogen can cause disease in different organs of the body. More than one disease can occur at a time. Symptoms (what the patient says, for example, a headache is called a symptom) and signs (what doctors see, such as blood pressure or blisters on the body) depend on the infected person's body system and the organisms involved. Almost all HIV-related diseases have fever as a symptom.

Originally, AIDS was defined as a group of rare fungal, viral, and parasitic infections, cancers, and some bacterial diseases that are seen in developed countries. In 1993, the CDC included tuberculosis, frequent bacterial pneumonia, and invasive cervical cancer (caused by the human papillomavirus) among the most life-threatening AIDS diseases in patients in poor and developing countries.

In the absence of antiretroviral therapy, the patient is susceptible to a wide range of infectious diseases. Eventually, the viral load in the patient's body increases greatly, and the CD4+ lymphocytes decrease drastically, rendering the body unable to fight any disease. That is how the patient dies. Treating only the opportunistic infections that afflict an HIV patient in contexts where antiretroviral therapy is not available may also improve survival for a few more years. This was the approach that doctors followed when drugs for HIV were not available or inaccessible.

The type of infections that occur in HIV patients correlates with the CD4+ lymphocyte count. In developing and poor countries, tuberculosis can affect patients at any time during the course of the disease. Tuberculosis can also occur in people with conditions that impair immune system function to some extent, such as malnutrition, aging, diabetes, and steroid use. The tuberculosis bacterium is more virulent. This is why many HIV patients in poor countries continue to be afflicted with tuberculosis, even though their CD4+ lymphocyte counts remain within the normal range for healthy individuals.

CD4+ Count and Disease Susceptibility: A Critical Link

The U.S. Centers for Disease Control and Prevention has called the disorder 'AIDS,' referring to certain life-threatening diseases that occur when the immune system of HIV sufferers is severely compromised, i.e., CD4+ lymphocytes are reduced to less than 200.

HIV-AIDS

When CD4+ lymphocytes are less than 200, they are prone to rare diseases like Coccidioidomycosis (lung disease), Invasive Cervical Cancer (caused by Human Papilloma Virus), Kaposi Sarcoma (caused by Human Herpes Virus 8), Progressive Multifocal Meningo Encephalitis (brain disease), *Pneumocystis jiroveci* pneumonia, *Toxoplasma* parasite infection of the brain, Histoplasmosis.

When CD4+ lymphocytes fall to less than 100 these patients become ill with oesophagus candidiasis (fungus infection of oesophagus), *Cryptococcus* neoformans meningitis, *Cryptosporidium* dysentery, *Cystoisosporidium* dysentery, severe herpes infection, bacillary angiomatosis.

When CD4+ lymphocytes are less than 50, rare diseases such as lymphoma (cancer) in the brain, cytomegalovirus infection in the eye, brain and lungs, and *Mycobacterium avium intracellular complex* in the lungs can occur. However, in communities where infectious diseases are prevalent, HIV sufferers are less likely to contract many of these diseases.

*Only one in a few hundred people with AIDS in India suffers from this type of pneumonia. Since the beginning, globally it has been the standard practice to give every patient diagnosed with HIV a drug to prevent *Pneumocystis* infection. Although the same is being followed in developing countries, the author of this book has never offered this preventive therapy. Due to this, not only a lot of trouble was avoided for the patients, but it was also possible to do without unnecessary expenditure.

**Kaposi sarcoma is very rare in India. The author of the book, who treated more than 6,000 HIV patients, diagnosed only one person with the disease over a period of 23 years.

10. HIV - AIDS Testing

Tests like ELISA, Western blot, and PCR confirm HIV.
Appropriate tests diagnose the various infections in AIDS.

When and Why HIV Testing is Recommended:

People infected with HIV usually consult a doctor with symptoms of an infectious disease, such as fever, diarrhoea, cough, and weight loss. In cases where doctors do not see the expected relief from the usual treatments, the patient is tested for HIV, taking into account some other factors. In developed countries, diseases that are seen in AIDS rarely occur in others. However, in developing and poor countries, including India, most of the infections that HIV patients fall ill with are the same as those that occur in others in the community. However, a small proportion of people who are infected with HIV suffer from some rare diseases. The symptoms and progression of these diseases are slightly different from those seen in people who are not infected with HIV. Therefore, the diagnosis of HIV/AIDS is a little more complicated.

HIV testing plays a crucial role in diagnosing HIV infection and preventing its transmission. Screening is recommended for all pregnant women to ensure early detection and treatment, which can significantly improve maternal and infant health outcomes. Additionally, individuals at increased risk of HIV infection, such as sex workers, transgender individuals, injecting drug users, and those diagnosed with sexually transmitted diseases, should be tested for HIV when they visit a healthcare facility. Doctors may also recommend HIV testing for other patients based on individual clinical judgment.

Diagnostic Challenges & Complexities in HIV/AIDS:

Diagnosing AIDS involves identifying both the HIV infection and any associated opportunistic infection/s. These infections occur because HIV weakens the immune system, making it harder for the body to fight off other pathogens. Doctors use various diagnostic methods specific to each suspected infectious disease. For example, if a patient has a cough, a chest X-ray, sputum analysis, and blood tests may be ordered.

Several types of HIV tests are available, each with its own advantages and limitations. Antigen and nucleic acid tests directly detect components of the HIV virus. Antigen tests can detect HIV infection relatively early, between 10 days and 4 weeks after infection, but they are not as widely available as antibody tests.

Antibody tests, which detect the body's immune response to HIV, are cost-effective, reliable, and widely available. However, it can take three to six weeks after infection for the body to produce detectable antibodies, known as the 'window period.' During this period, antibody tests may not accurately diagnose HIV infection.

By understanding the different types of HIV tests and their appropriate uses, healthcare providers can ensure a timely and accurate diagnosis of HIV infection and provide appropriate care and treatment.

HIV Testing Methods: A Range of Options for Detection

HIV antigen tests: Polymerase chain reaction (PCR) is an expensive and complex test used to detect HIV antigens. A proviral DNA test can indicate a positive result from 10 days after HIV infection. To diagnose mother-to-child transmission of HIV infection, it is carried out on infants born to HIV-infected women, from the age of 14 days to 21 days. If the baby is breastfed, it is done once every 3 months for the infant and three months after the cessation of breastfeeding.

Even when HIV is positive in antigen tests, it is confirmed by antibody testing. In cases of acute infections, the disease is sometimes diagnosed with antigen tests. P24 antigen detection tests are used to detect HIV infection from two weeks to four weeks after infection. However, when the patient's body releases antibodies between 4 weeks to 8 weeks, the P24 antigen level decreases drastically. Therefore, antigen tests performed after 8 weeks are more likely to show a false negative result.

Antibody tests, which detect the body's immune response to HIV, are cost-effective, reliable, and widely available. Several types of antibody tests exist, including ELISA, DOT ELISA, and agglutination assays. Various companies market these tests under a variety of brand names, such as Trident, Determine, HIV Spot, Insti, Immunoconb, CombAids, Retrotec, RetroQuick, and Capillus. These tests work by detecting antibodies produced by B lymphocytes, a type of white blood cell, in response to HIV infection. While antibody tests are generally accurate, they may show negative results during the window period, which is the time between infection and when the body produces detectable antibodies. This period typically lasts three to six weeks, but in some cases, it can take longer. It is important to note that during the window period, a person can still transmit HIV to others even if their antibody test is negative.

In addition to presenting infectious disease, HIV infection should also be diagnosed. The enzyme-linked immunosorbent assay (ELISA or EIA) is the most used test to diagnose HIV infection. For individual tests, the test form is called 'Cassette ELISA,' in which each patient is tested separately. The Tridot test is a popular cassette Elisa test. Surveys and blood banks use microwell ELISA to test a large number of blood samples, 96 at a time.

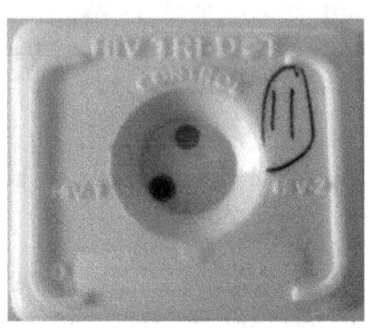 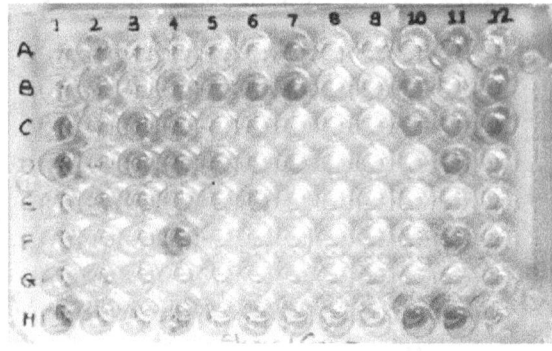

Cassette Elisa Test   *Microwell Elisa Test*

Tests to detect HIV with saliva testing have also become available. And they were not very popular.

HIV tests can rarely show a false positive, that showing positive result in the absence of infection. Therefore, HIV infection can be confirmed by performing a sophisticated modern test called Western Blot. A western blot test looks for three different antigens (parts) of HIV. Three simple tests dependent on different antigens can also be done at a low cost to confirm HIV infection.

The ELISA and Western blot tests are based on the antibodies (proteins) produced by the human body when it is infected with the virus, rather than the virus itself or the virus components. The most commonly used ELISA tests employ major component(s) of HIV to detect antibodies produced by the patient's body against it. The Western blot test detects the antibodies produced by the patient's body against the three principal components of HIV: Gag (group antigen), Pol (polymerase), and Env (envelope).

Recently, ELISA tests (third generation) have become available that detect the components (antigens) of HIV along with antibodies. It is possible to detect HIV infection within 15 days of infection, HIV infection can be detected. HIV infection can be detected.

Diagnosing HIV in Children:

However, even if HIV is not transmitted from the mother to the child born to the infected woman, HIV antibodies can still be transmitted. In this case, either the antibody detection test or the western blot may be positive. Antibodies from the mother vanish by the time the child is 18 months old. Antibody tests then confirm HIV infection.

During the window period, there are no antibodies to HIV. In such cases, tests that directly detect the HIV virus or its components need to be performed.

Therefore, when choosing a diagnostic test for HIV, consider all relevant factors.

Assessing Immune System Health and Viral Activity:

AIDS tests are tests to determine the number of lymphocytes and the quantity of the virus (viral load). Doctors interpret the results of AIDS tests based on the patient's symptoms, severity of the disease, and response to treatment.

The CD4+ (T-helper) lymphocyte count test is done to assess the damage inflicted on the immune system by HIV. We perform this test using a flow cytometer device. A CD4+ lymphocyte count of less than 200 is considered to indicate advanced disease. Such patients can easily be vulnerable to various infectious diseases.

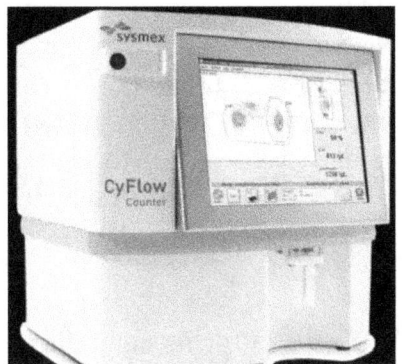

In the early days, the number of CD4+ cells less than 200 was considered AIDS. However, it is a parameter used to collect data. Although the number of CD4+ cells is very low, many patients recover with antiretroviral therapy. The HIV viral load (quantitative PCR) test is done to determine the activity and severity of the virus. PCR tests are performed with a thermal cycler / thermocycler device.

Flow cytometer that measures. CD4+ and CD8 lymphocytes

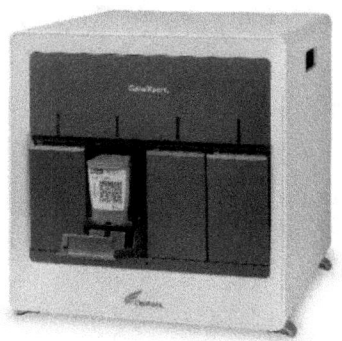
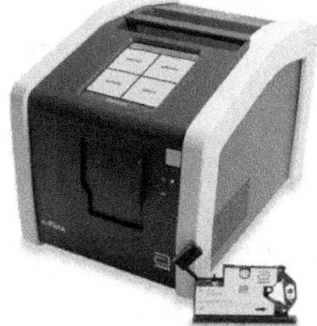

Thermal Cyclers for HIV Viral Load Test

There are thousands to millions of HIV copies per millilitre of blood in any untreated condition. Shortly after treatment, the virus becomes contained. The virus replication is halted in such a way that it cannot be detected in tests. This is called an undetectable viral load. However, copies of the HIV gene remain in the DNA of the patient's CD4+ cells, macrophages, and a few other cells. If the treatment is stopped, the virus can replicate again, and the viral load bounces back in a short time.

Antigen-quantitative PCR tests are done to determine the viral load of HIV. This test is done to detect changes in viral load due to antiretroviral therapy and to determine the severity of the disease. A pro-viral DNA viral phenotyping test can help determine the appropriate medication for the patient when medication changes are necessary. The 1996 definition of AIDS defines it as having more than 30,000 copies of the virus per millilitre of blood. Now it is not taken into consideration.

HIV Genotyping and Phenotyping:

HIV genotyping and phenotyping are crucial laboratory techniques employed to analyse the genetic makeup and characteristics of the human immunodeficiency virus (HIV) in individual patients. These tests play a vital role in guiding treatment decisions and optimizing antiretroviral therapy.

Genotyping involves sequencing the viral genome to identify specific mutations that may confer resistance to certain antiretroviral drugs. This is typically achieved through polymerase chain reaction (PCR) amplification of the viral RNA, followed by DNA sequencing techniques like Sanger sequencing or next-generation sequencing. By comparing the patient's viral sequence to a reference strain, healthcare providers can pinpoint mutations associated with drug resistance. Phenotyping, on the other hand, takes a more direct approach. It involves growing the patient's viral strain in cell cultures and exposing it to various antiretroviral drugs. The virus's ability to replicate in the presence of these drugs is then measured, providing a quantitative assessment of drug resistance. Phenotyping assays may use recombinant virus particles or clinical isolates from the patient.

Window Period: Limitations of Antibody Tests:

In the window period, since there are no antibodies, HIV or its components must be identified. For this, a polymerase chain reaction (PCR) test is performed. Tests to detect antibodies after the window period (after 3 months): ELISA, Western Blot, etc.

Antibody tests are not useful to diagnose the disease in infants of HIV-positive mothers. Because antibodies are passed from mother to baby, antibody tests cannot diagnose the disease. A PCR test should be done. Antibody testing should be done after 18 months of age.

AIDS severity tests: CD4+ (T-helper) lymphocyte count tests, virus quantity PCR tests. The test for detecting HIV infection is called qualitative PCR, and the viral load test for prescribing treatment is called quantitative PCR.

11. Treatment of HIV - AIDS

Expensive treatment can significantly improve HIV patients' longevity and quality of life. Treatment of associated infectious diseases can prolong their lives for many years.

Many people believe that AIDS is a deadly disease with no cure. Researchers have studied this single microbial agent more extensively than any other. Despite this in-depth understanding, no curative treatment is available to date. Medical research has led to the discovery of many drugs that are active against HIV. However, they have not been able to completely cure the HIV infection.

Let us look at what a complete cure means. The bacterium *Salmonella typhi*, for example, causes typhoid. For its treatment, Ciprofloxacin, Azithromycin, Ceftriaxone, and other medicines are currently available. Giving these medications to the patient destroys and eliminates the typhoid bacteria from the body. After successful treatment, there is no trace of Salmonella in the patient's blood. However, this is not the case with HIV. HIV can enter the patient's CD4+ lymphocytes, as well as some other reservoirs, and escape the medication. No currently available HIV treatment has eliminated the virus from a patient's body. The treatments halt viral replication, and the virus can be grown from the patient's blood by culture. This means that the HIV virus remains dormant in the patient's blood and is not eliminated.

There is currently no cure for HIV/AIDS. After HIV infection, the virus replicates and grows, and the number of CD4+ lymphocytes gradually decreases. The patient becomes vulnerable to various infections. However, by preventing replication at different stages, we can contain the virus replication and growth. Antiretroviral drugs work against HIV. To date, there are 34 agents of anti-HIV drugs and two agents that are boosters. Although some of these drugs were effective, they were withdrawn due to adverse effects. At present, 22 different drugs and two booster agents are available.

Some of the infected cells remain dormant. These are called memory cells or latent reservoir cells. Typically, any infection causes some changes in the shape and topology of the infected cells. As a result of these changes, the body's immune system recognizes them and destroys the infected cells. Because HIV does not replicate in these cells, there are no changes in the cells that the immune system can detect.

Some of the HIV-infected cells become lytic, productive cells. HIV is constantly growing in these cells. CD4+ lymphocytes, which play a key role in the immune system, produce chemicals that stimulate other cells when a pathogen enters the body. But in such a case, these HIV-infected lytic cells make up the components of the virus, eventually producing the virus particles (virions).

To develop drugs for any infectious disease, one must first know the stages of the growth cycle of the pathogen that causes the disease. Appropriate molecules (drugs) interrupt or interfere with various stages of the replication cycle, thereby preventing the growth of pathogens. The human immunodeficiency virus (HIV), responsible for AIDS, attaches itself to a protein known as CD4+ on specific cells to infect humans. Next, with the help of chemokine receptors (co-receptors) named CCR5 and CXCR4, the virus strips the envelope, and the capsid containing the genes and enzymes of the virus enters the human cell. Then an enzyme called reverse transcriptase of the virus uses the mechanism of the human cell to make a copy of the DNA from the RNA of the virus. Next, complementary DNA copy of the virus is generated to make double-stranded DNA. Later, this double-stranded DNA is integrated into the human DNA with the help of an enzyme called 'integrase.' Now the virus is permanently part of the human body. Activation of the infected CD4+ lymphocytes produces the virus's proteins. The protease enzyme cleaves and matures the long viral proteins to form a functional virus. The virus molecule makes pores in the wall of the CD4+ cell and makes an envelope out of the lymphocyte membrane, allowing the virus cells (virions) to escape. In this way, the CD4+ cell lyses and dies.

Drug Resistance and Combination Therapy in Infectious Diseases:

Many infectious diseases are treated with a single drug. However, some diseases are not sufficiently controlled by a single drug. Such diseases require treatment with a combination of more than one drug. At the beginning of the introduction of a new drug, most infectious diseases caused by pathogens are usually treatable with a single drug for some time, often a few years or decades. However, over time, due to evolutionary pressures and natural selection, some pathogens can develop mechanisms to survive and replicate in the presence of the drug, leading to drug resistance. When drug resistance emerges, the disease may become more difficult to treat with the single drug alone. In such circumstances, combination therapy, which involves using two or more drugs with different mechanisms of action, is often employed to inhibit the growth of the drug-resistant pathogen more effectively. Treatment for tuberculosis involves four drugs, as many people are aware. Antibiotic resistance is a major problem facing the world today. In other words, diseases that were previously treatable with drugs are now resistant to any available drugs.

Targeting Different Stages of the HIV Lifecycle:

Nucleoside and nucleotide reverse transcriptase inhibitors are drugs that first became available for the treatment of HIV in 1987. Protease inhibitors began with Saquinavir in 1995. The category of non-nucleoside reverse transcriptase inhibitors began with Efavirenz in 1996. Enfuvertide (T20), the only injectable drug in the

Fusion / Attachment Inhibitors class, has been available since 2003. used rarely. Maraviroc belongs to the chemokine co-receptor (CCR5) antagonist class and was introduced in 2007.

For the treatment of HIV, drugs that are active at different stages of the replication cycle of the virus are used. Two nucleoside reverse transcriptase inhibitors have been the backbone of three-drug antiretroviral therapy since 1996. In other words, they combine with another class of drugs. However, integrase-strand transfer inhibitors (INSTIs) are currently replacing the NRTI backbone. Currently, combinations of other drugs with integrase inhibitors are the mainstay of HIV treatment. Since late 2022, a two-drug combination has also been used in previously untreated (treatment-naive) patients. Dolutegravir and Lamivudine A combination is recommended for newly diagnosed patients. Currently, the only available injection treatment is Cabotegravir and Rilpivirine, is a combination of two drugs.
*

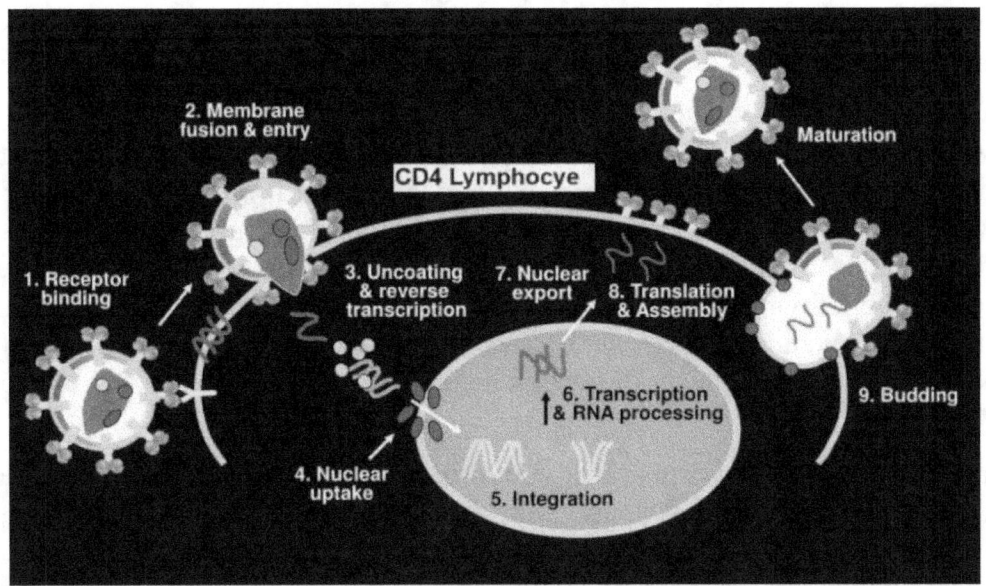

Stages in HIV Replication

Antiretroviral Drugs:

With the introduction of Zidovudine for treatment of AIDS in March 1987, patients' health improved within a few weeks, and everyone was jubilant that treatment for HIV finally became available. However, the CD4+ lymphocyte count began to decline after six months in the patients who initially improved. After almost two years of taking Zidovudine, the health of many patients had deteriorated. Some patients who were on Zidovudine and worsened over time were given the drug Didanosine, which was available since October 1991, and with the two-drug combination, their condition improved.

HAART: Game Changer in HIV Management

A new chapter in the treatment of AIDS began in 1995 with triple drug therapy with Saquinavir, a protease enzyme inhibitor. Treatment with two nucleoside inhibitors and one protease inhibitor stopped the HIV's growth, resulting in a low viral load in the patient's blood that modern PCR equipment could not detect. In 1996, at the 11th International AIDS Conference in Vancouver, Canada, Dr. David Ho, and his colleagues presented the results of their ground-breaking research showing that a combination of three drugs can provide great relief from AIDS. In September of the same year, the U.S. Centers for Disease Control and Prevention (CDC) announced three drug combination Highly Active Antiretroviral Treatment (HAART) guidelines for the treatment of AIDS.

Classification of antiretroviral drugs:

They can be divided into six categories. Reverse transcriptase inhibitors: Soon after HIV capsid is released into CD4+ lymphocyte, the enzyme reverse transcriptase makes a DNA copy of viral RNA genes as a prerequisite for entering human DNA. Reverse transcriptase inhibitors interfere in this process. This prevents the further steps in replication of HIV. These include nucleoside / nucleotide reverse transcriptase inhibitors and non-nucleoside reverse transcriptase inhibitors.

1. Nucleoside/Nucleotide reverse transcriptase inhibitors (NRTIs): were the first drugs available to treat HIV. These prevent the DNA chain from elongating when the reverse transcriptase enzyme tries to make a copy of the viral RNA into DNA. These are called chain terminators. NRTIs include Abacavir, Emtricitabine, Lamivudine, Tenofovir disoproxil, Tenofovir alafenamide (a newer formulation), Zidovudine, Stavudine, Didanosine, and Zalcitabine. The availability of Didanosine* and Zalcitabine has ceased, while the phase-out of Stavudine** is also underway.

2. Non-nucleoside reverse transcriptase inhibitors (NNRTIs) directly inhibit the activity of the reverse transcriptase enzyme. This class includes Efavirenz, Nevirapine, Doravirine, Delaviridine, Etravirine, and others. Rilpivirine, from this class, is currently used in combination with Cabotegravir as a long-acting injectable treatment.

3. Integrase Strand Transfer Inhibitors (INSTIs) act on the integrase enzyme, which helps integrate the HIV genetic material into the human DNA after the reverse transcriptase enzyme converts the viral RNA into DNA. INSTI drugs block the action of the HIV integrase enzyme, preventing the integration of viral DNA into the patient's DNA. Drugs in this category include Dolutegravir, Raltegravir, Bictegravir, and Elvitegravir. Cabotegravir, an injectable formulation from the same group, is now popular as a long-acting drug. A drug called Cobicistat is used to boost the levels of Elvitegravir.

4. Protease inhibitors: HIV virus proteins are produced as large molecules within infected human cells and require cleavage by an enzyme called protease for viral maturation. Protease inhibitors inhibit the growth of HIV by blocking this protease enzyme. This group includes Atazanavir, Lopinavir, Darunavir, Saquinavir,

Indinavir, Fosamprenavir, Tipranavir, and Nelfinavir. The drug Ritonavir from this group is used as a booster to enhance the activity of other protease inhibitors.

5. Capsid Inhibitors: The nucleocapsid is a cone-shaped structure that encapsulates HIV's genetic material and enzymes. Capsid inhibitors are a new class of drugs that prevent the formation of this nucleocapsid. Lenacapavir, a drug belonging to the capsid inhibitor class, became available in late 2022. In the future, these capsid inhibitors will likely play a major role in the treatment of HIV.

6. Other drugs include Attachment and post-attachment inhibitors:

Attachment and Post-Attachment Inhibitors: These drugs block the attachment of HIV to the human CD4+ protein of human cells and the subsequent stages of viral entry.

Fusion Inhibitors: Enfuvirtide (an injectable drug) CCR5 antagonists: maraviroc (a CCR5 receptor antagonist) Post-Attachment Inhibitors: Ibalizumab (a monoclonal antibody).

From Low CD4+ Count to Test and Treat

Monitoring Treatment with Viral Load and CD4+ Count:

HIV can make frequent changes in its genotype (mutates) to become resistant to the drugs used for treatment. Thus, even if one or both drugs initially reduce the viral load for some time (which is determined by the viral load), the HIV strains in the patient's body soon become resistant to those drugs. Therefore, multi-drug treatment for HIV is a must. Three or more antiretroviral drugs should be given simultaneously. The first HIV standard treatment guidelines, issued in 1996, recommended that antiretroviral therapy be started when the CD4+ lymphocyte count per microlitre of blood is less than 200 and/or there are 30,000 copies of the virus per millilitre. Antiretroviral therapy should be initiated if the patient is diagnosed with an opportunistic infection indicative of AIDS, irrespective of the viral load or CD4+ cell count.

As of 2009, the World Health Organization (WHO) recommended initiating antiretroviral therapy if there were more than 30,000 virus copies per millilitre of the patient's blood or if the CD4+ lymphocyte count was less than 350 cells/mm^3. In 2013, it was recommended to start treatment if the number of CD4+ cells was less than 500 cells/ml. Several studies have shown that starting treatment before significant damage to the immune system helps prevent patients from contracting various infections. Since 2015, the guidelines have recommended that patients start treatment on the day of HIV diagnosis, irrespective of the CD4+ lymphocyte count. This is known as the "test and treat" approach.

Newer Drugs:

Several new antiretroviral molecules are currently in development, targeting different stages of the HIV life cycle. Among entry inhibitors, Albuvirtide is approved in China but not in the US or Europe. In the nucleoside reverse transcriptase translocation inhibitor (NRTTI) class, Islatravir and MK-8527 are showing promise with their novel mechanism of action but are still under investigation. Non-nucleoside reverse transcriptase inhibitors (NNRTIs) like Elsulfavirine (approved in Russia and neighbouring countries), ACC0007 (not yet approved), and S-365598 (not approved) are being evaluated for their efficacy against drug-resistant HIV strains. Lenacapavir, a capsid inhibitor, is approved in the US and Europe for heavily treatment-experienced individuals with multi-drug resistant HIV-1. Broadly neutralizing antibodies (bNAbs) such as VRac 01/LS, VRC 07/LS, GS-6423, GS-2872, and NGLS are being explored for their potential to neutralize a wide range of HIV strains, but none are currently approved. Additionally, maturation inhibitors like GSK254 and GSK927 are likely in the early stages of research and development, with none currently approved. These diverse molecules hold promise for improving HIV treatment options, particularly for drug-resistant cases and long-acting formulations.

HIV/AIDS is now a Chronic Manageable Condition:

Response to treatment: Untreated HIV patients typically have between 100,000 and one million copies of the viral load per millilitre of blood. HIV stops replicating and growing within a few weeks of starting treatment. The level, which can be detected by state-of-the-art equipment, is reduced to no more than 20 copies per millilitre. This is called an undetectable viral load. And with effective treatment, the life expectancy of these patients reaches a near-normal level.

Highly active antiretroviral therapy (HAART), or simply antiretroviral therapy (ART), involves the use of three or more antiretroviral drugs simultaneously. Several factors need to be considered before starting treatment, including the choice of drug combination. These drugs are effective only in certain combinations. After starting HIV treatment, patients should continue to take medications regularly, similar to taking medicines for chronic conditions like diabetes and high blood pressure. Because HIV research is expensive, HIV drugs are generally expensive.

In developed countries, HIV treatment often involves polypharmacy, where multiple individual antiretroviral drugs are taken as separate pills. This is due to the availability of various products from different innovator pharmaceutical companies. In contrast, in developing countries, fixed-dose combination (FDC) pills containing two or three antiretroviral drugs in a single tablet are more commonly used. The requirement of taking multiple pills daily for HIV treatment in developed countries may lead to apprehension, guilt, or stigma for some individuals living with HIV, as it serves as a constant reminder of their HIV-positive status.

The development of newer antiretroviral molecules is focusing on less frequent administration in addition to treating multiple drug-resistant HIV patients.

Challenges in Resource - Limited Settings:

However, with ART, the fear of AIDS in Western countries has completely subsided. Within two to eight weeks of starting this treatment, the patient achieves a minimal quantity of HIV in the blood. With an increase in the number of CD4+ lymphocytes, one can regain health and lead a normal life for an extended period of time. In late 1996, the U.S. Department of Health removed HIV/AIDS from the list of life-threatening diseases and placed it in the category of chronic manageable diseases. However, even without expensive antiretroviral therapy, life expectancy can be extended by a few years if appropriate treatment is provided for the opportunistic infections that afflict these patients.

UNAIDS (Joint United Nations Programme on AIDS) in collaboration with international agencies like the World Health Organization, the Global Fund for AIDS TB and Malaria (GFATM), Australian Aid (AUAID), British Aid (DFID), US Government Assistance (USAID), German Aid (GTZ), the Bill and Melinda Gates Foundation (BMGF), the Clinton Foundation, and Médecins Sans Frontières are providing HIV medicines free of cost to poor countries. However, the use of antiretrovirals has not improved the health of patients in poor developing countries to the extent that it has in developed countries. The reason for this may be the lack of adequate expertise and awareness among doctors in these countries.

Evolution of HIV treatment:

Since 1996, a triple-drug combination antiretroviral treatment known as highly active antiretroviral therapy (HAART) has become the standard of care in HIV management. HAART consists of a combination of three or more antiretroviral drugs from different classes, targeting various stages of the HIV life cycle to maximally suppress the virus and reduce the risk of drug resistance. Typical HAART regimens involve two nucleoside reverse transcriptase inhibitors (NRTIs) combined with either a protease inhibitor, a non-nucleoside reverse transcriptase inhibitor (NNRTI), or an integrase strand transfer inhibitor (INSTI). By inhibiting HIV replication through different mechanisms, HAART can substantially reduce viral load, slow disease progression, and improve long-term prognosis more effectively than single-drug therapy.

Despite the effectiveness of antiretroviral therapy, HIV patients experience sustained inflammation and immune activation, increasing their risk for developing lifestyle diseases like cardiovascular disease, diabetes, and certain cancers. As a result, the incidence of these comorbidities is higher among HIV patients compared to the general population. While the life expectancy of HIV patients has significantly improved and is nearing that of the general population, it is still not on par due to the chronic inflammatory state and associated complications. Moreover, the management of these comorbidities in HIV patients is complicated by potential drug interactions between antiretroviral medications and treatments for other diseases, posing challenges in achieving optimal therapeutic outcomes and requiring careful monitoring and adjustment of drug regimens.***

* It was withdrawn due to the adverse effect of pancreatitis, which is seen more in countries where liquor consumption is a part of people's lives and cultures. But Didanosine and Stavudine are good drugs for patients in India, according to the author.

**The author has been treating most of his HIV patients with two-drug combinations since the start of his professional practice in 2000. The author presented his study on two-drug antiretroviral therapy at the 2004 International Symposium on HIV and Emerging Infectious Diseases (ISHEID) in Toulon, France.

*** The guidelines for HIV treatment mainly come from studies conducted at tertiary care centres, which typically involve treatment-experienced patients. Hence, these guidelines usually recommend newer antiretroviral molecules. However, the majority of patients in developing countries have either never been exposed to antiretroviral therapy or have had minimal exposure. The author suggests formulating a different set of guidelines using two-drug antiretroviral combinations to address the treatment needs of these previously untreated or minimally treated patients in developing countries.

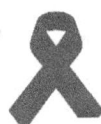

12. Two-Drug Antiretroviral Therapy

The two-drug treatment regimen that Dr Yanamadala has been offering since 2000 has found its place in treatment guidelines after two decades.

Global Landscape of HIV Treatment and Research: The global response to AIDS has been marked by disparities in research and access to treatment. While studies and research are vital for shedding light on new insights and findings, a critical gap exists in basic research for diseases prevalent in developing nations. AIDS, a major public health concern in India, exemplifies this disparity.

In the early years, the CDC guidelines for AIDS diagnosis and treatment were widely adopted globally. These guidelines emphasized frequent, often expensive, testing and costly medical treatment. The financial burden associated with these approaches prompted a search for more affordable and accessible treatment options within communities.

The Evolution of Antiretroviral Therapy: Zidovudine, the first antiretroviral drug to treat AIDS, was introduced in 1987, followed by Didanosine in 1991. By 1995, six antiretroviral drugs, including Saquinavir, were available. In September 1996, the CDC standardised HIV treatment with a three-drug combination. As new medications emerged, different combinations became possible, leading to the prescription of newer three-drug regimens. European AIDS treatment guidelines, released shortly after, also advocated for a three-drug combination as the standard treatment.

Dr. Yanamadala's Approach and Its Rationale: When Dr. Yanamadala began his career in Kakinada as the first exclusive HIV Physician in Andhra Pradesh, India, in 2000, four antiretroviral drugs (Zidovudine, Lamivudine, Stavudine, and Nevirapine) were available in India. This allowed for two three-drug combinations. However, based on his research and experience, Dr. Yanamadala concluded that a two-drug regimen was often more effective for newly diagnosed patients. The rationale behind Dr. Yanamadala's approach rests on the observation that newly introduced antiretroviral drugs are often added to patients whose previous treatment regimens have failed. While a three-drug combination is recommended for better disease control, the newest drug in a three-drug regimen may be the only one working to its full potential. The virus can develop resistance to the two older drugs, rendering them partially or completely ineffective. In essence, although three drugs are being administered, only two may be effectively working.

Dr. Yanamadala's Findings and Early Advocacy: Dr. Yanamadala's research has demonstrated that a two-drug regimen can be effective for newly diagnosed HIV patients. This approach challenges the long-held recommendation for three-drug combinations, offering a potential solution for more affordable and accessible treatment in resource-constrained settings.

In 2004, Dr. Yanamadala presented a research abstract at the 13th International Symposium on HIV and Emerging Infectious Diseases (ISHEID) in Toulon, France, proposing a novel approach to HIV treatment in resource-limited settings. His research focused on the unique situation in countries like India, where access to antiretroviral therapy was extremely limited at the time, meaning the virus was largely "treatment-naïve" and potentially more susceptible to various drug regimens.

Dr. Yanamadala hypothesized that initiating treatment with two appropriate drugs simultaneously could achieve a potent synergistic effect, effectively suppressing HIV replication. This two-drug approach offered several advantages: lower cost, simpler administration, potentially improved adherence, and keeping future options open.

However, this cost-effective strategy was not commercially attractive to the pharmaceutical industry and therefore received little attention or research funding. Despite this, Dr. Yanamadala continued to advocate for the two-drug regimens. Over time, others began to explore similar ideas.

Landmark Shift: Two-Drug Regimens become options in HIV Management

Finally, in 2019, research emerged supporting the efficacy of two-drug combination HIV treatment in newly diagnosed patients. This culminated in a landmark shift in 2022, when both the CDC and the European AIDS Clinical Society (EACS) updated their guidelines to include two-drug regimens (Dolutegravir plus Lamivudine) as a viable option for newly diagnosed HIV patients. Further illustrating this paradigm shift, the first long-term injectable treatment for HIV, approved in December 2022, also comprised a combination of two drugs: Rilpivirine and Cabotegravir.

This journey towards the acceptance of two-drug HIV therapy as an option underscores the importance of continued research and advocacy, even for ideas that initially face resistance or lack commercial appeal. Ultimately, such efforts can lead to significant advancements in healthcare, particularly for vulnerable populations in resource-limited settings. It should be noted that the "treatment-naïve" mentioned in Dr. Yanamadala's 2004 research and the "newly diagnosed" in the current HIV treatment guidelines are essentially the same.

A Decade Ahead: Proving Effectiveness of Two-Drug Treatment: Dr. Yanamadala Murali Krishna has managed his patients with a thorough and in-depth understanding of AIDS. He has made two notable contributions: advocating for and implementing two-drug HIV treatment regimens and making HIV treatment accessible to the poor without relying heavily on diagnostic tests, supporting 6,000 families over a period of 23 years.

- PP 4.38 Natural Treatment for HIV/AIDS
  Schelonka EP. Good News Medical Clinic, Belize City, Belize - Central America

- PP 4.39 Vivre avec le Secret du VIH et des Multithérapies pour un Groupe de Femmes Montréalaises
  Trottier G, Massie L, Toupin I, Fernet M, Otis J, Pelletier R, Bastien R, Josy Lévy J, Samson J, Boucher M, Lapointe N, Harerimana M et Rateau M. Québec - Canada

- PP 4.40 Two-drug ART in Treatment Naïve HIV-infected Persons in Resource-limited Setting: 2-year study
  Yanamadala VMKR. Association of People Against AIDS, Kakinada, Andhra Pradesh - India

- PP 4.41 The Dissociation Between Immunologic and Virologic Response to HAART
  Pesic I, Salemovic D, Ranin J, Zerjav S, Jevtovic Dj. The Institute of Infectious and Tropical Diseases, Belgrade - Serbia & Montenegro

- PP 4.42 Utilization of HIV Post Exposure Prophylaxis Among Health Care Workers in Selected Health Institutions In Nairobi
  Maina JW, Wasunna MK, Orago AS, Okelo RO.Kenyatta University, Nairobi - Kenya

Dr. Yanamadala was at least a decade and a half ahead of the global medical community in advocating for and implementing two-drug HIV treatment regimens. His work has led to significant advancements in healthcare for vulnerable populations in resource-limited settings, demonstrating the power of vision, perseverance, and a commitment to improving the lives of others.

Scan the QR code for the ISHEID Abstract Book link.

Looking Forward: Dr. Yanamadala Murali Krishna, an HIV medical practitioner from Kakinada city, solely managed all his patients and made HIV treatment accessible to the poor without relying heavily on diagnostic tests, supporting 6,000 families over a period of 23 years. He has made two notable contributions with a thorough and in-depth understanding of AIDS. Several other new findings have been made, providing patients with effective treatment. Dr. Yanamadala Murali Krishna was at least a decade and a half ahead of the global medical community in advocating for and implementing two-drug HIV treatment regimens.

13. Fight for the Rights of AIDS-Affected

The AIDS patients were subjected to severe agony as they were looked down on by society. The struggles of victims and rights activists have brought them some relief from stigma.

Early Misunderstandings and Discrimination:

AIDS was first identified in gay men. Later, recreational injection-drug users were also diagnosed with AIDS. At that time, the community had strong feelings against these groups. The people saw it as God's punishment. There are many social and cultural barriers to talking about this disease. As a result, there were not enough public awareness programs and research on the disease in its early days. The victims of this disease have faced severe discrimination and a lack of access to treatment.

Within a short period of time, it became known that HIV can be transmitted from one person to another through body fluids and blood. The disease is mainly spread through sex. However, the deaths of sexually active youth due to this disease have alarmed everyone. In the early days, this disease caused great panic in the whole of society and even among doctors. At one time in history, AIDS created the worst terror that 'smallpox' caused, which claimed the lives of about 20 out of 100 people and left many more disfigured. Initially, the hospitals used to burn the beds and linen of patients who died of AIDS. Ambulances carrying patients were also torched in some unusual cases. In the early years of the epidemic, doctors and hospital staff wore special astronaut-style outfits to serve these patients. Now, after the emergence of COVID, such single-use PPE kits are familiar to everyone.

In recent times, governments, the science world, the medical world, and civil society have responded strongly to fight COVID. Although COVID can infect everyone, there is still a possibility that a huge number of people will die. A prompt response could greatly mitigate the tragedy and fatalities. The main reason for this is that COVID disease is related to the whole of society. But AIDS is not like that. It is a matter of small groups living separately, away from society. At the time, society's disapproval of these groups and their perceived inferiority complex was a barrier to assessing the severity and extent of the disease. The government's insufficient funding during the first two or three years of the disease led to an estimated loss of at least 1,000,000 lives. Politicians and civil society were not magnanimous enough to show interest in the disease.

Fighting for Recognition and Rights: AIDS survivor and activist Cleve Jones started the 'Names Project,' the AIDS Memorial Quilt, in November 1985. It is a powerful, poignant memorial to commemorate the lives of people who have died from AIDS-related illnesses. The idea was to remember those who died of AIDS through a quilt that was part of a middle-class American family. The project, which has become the world's largest community folk art piece, weighs 54 tons as of 2020. Jones, along with several others, founded the San Francisco AIDS Foundation in 1983, which has grown into one of the largest and most effective legal aid organizations empowering people with AIDS in the United States. Because of the demonstrations and fights about AIDS, mostly from the gay community, it was considered by the political elite and the public as a gay disease.

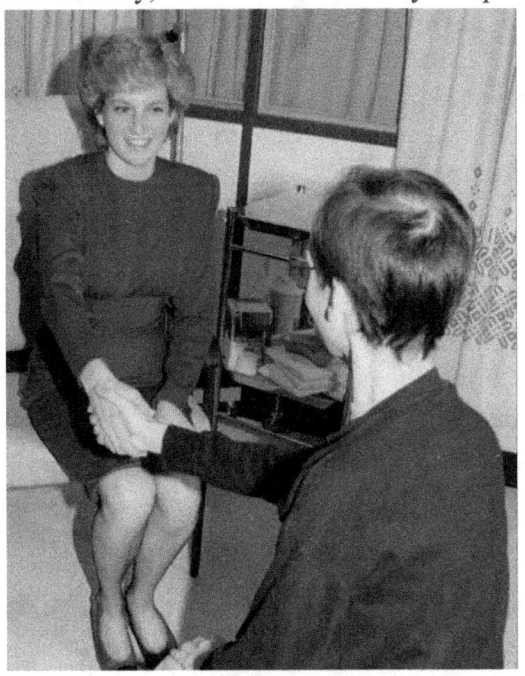

On April 9, 1987, Diana, Princess of Wales, opened the Broderip ward at the Middle Sex Hospital in London, dedicated to AIDS patients. She interacted with nine HIV patients in the hospital and shook hands with them. This greatly helped to change society's previous practice of exclusion and untouchability towards AIDS patients. Until then, no matter how much the government, the health sector, and the media campaigned to support AIDS patients against discrimination, the response was poor. The public's perception of Princess Diana came from the public's love and worship, which changed people's attitudes.

President Ronald Reagan pronounced the term AIDS in 1987, six years after the disease was discovered. It was not until the death of actor Rock Hudson that he was diagnosed with AIDS. Actor Rock Hudson died of AIDS in October 1985. AIDS got public attention. Elizabeth Taylor, co-star of Rock Hudson, established the American Foundation for AIDS Research (amfAR) with funding from Hudson Property. In the history of the AIDS epidemic, amfAR has had a big impact. Subsequently, Ryan White, a 13-year-old who frequently received factor VIII concentrates for haemophilia treatment, contracted AIDS and faced denial of school admission. He strongly protested discrimination against AIDS victims. He advocated for the equal rights of all AIDS victims and the respect of their rights.

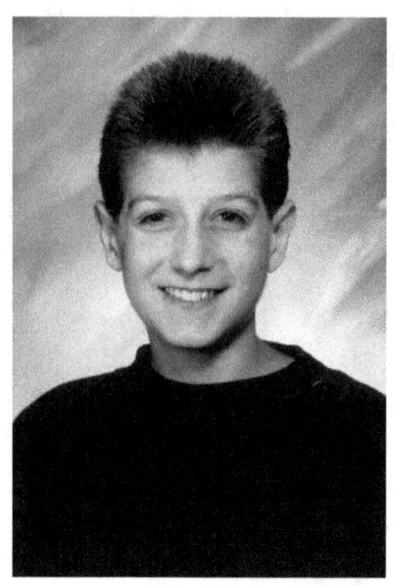
Ryan White

Despite not being homosexual, American basketball player Magic Johnson was diagnosed with AIDS. Cuban MTV star Pedro Zamora has campaigned extensively for the rights of AIDS victims.

Due to the fact that the disease of AIDS is found more in those who take injection drugs, many people do not even come forward to donate blood because of the widespread misconception that this disease can also be transmitted by the needle pierced while donating blood.

There have been several incidents where houses of AIDS patients have been set on fire. Since the government's contribution to the fight against AIDS was not great, the victims themselves formed groups and helped each other. End-of-life patients were nursed by fellow patients. Fellow patients also performed funerals for those who died of the disease. By the end of 1986, more than 24,000 Americans had died of AIDS.

The National Institutes of Health found in 1986 that AZT (azidothymidine, now known as Zidovudine), originally intended for cancer but abandoned due to unsatisfactory results, could improve the health of AIDS patients. This discovery united AIDS patients. However, demand for the expedited approval of the drug was widespread among AIDS patients. The government agencies will have to go through scrutiny and research to grant such permissions. It is a very time-consuming affair. It can take years, sometimes decades. The relief with azidothymidine has united thousands of people who were already at risk of dying from AIDS and their families. A massive campaign was launched to make this medicine available to everyone as soon as possible. In March 1987, the U.S. government approved AZT for use in HIV treatment for the shortest time in history. Thus, a new process of rapid access to medicines in the medical field began with AIDS. Following this precedent, research and trials swiftly introduced the COVID-19 vaccine. Initially, the cost of treatment with this drug ranged from 8,000 to ten thousand dollars per year. Although thousands of people need this drug, most of them are not able to afford such a cost. There was a massive movement by AIDS patients to make this medicine available to everyone at an affordable price.

Organizations and Individuals Making a Difference: New York activists Larry Kramer and Peter Staley founded the AIDS Coalition to Unleash Power (ACT-UP) in March 1987. This is the first time in history that patients with a single disease are fighting for treatment access. On September 14, 1989, Peter Staley, along with six other activists, entered the New York Stock Exchange to protest producer Burroughs Welcome for lowering AZT prices. The police arrested them and produced them in court. During the hearing of the case, the judge hailed the activists as heroes. The activists have reduced prices by 20 percent.

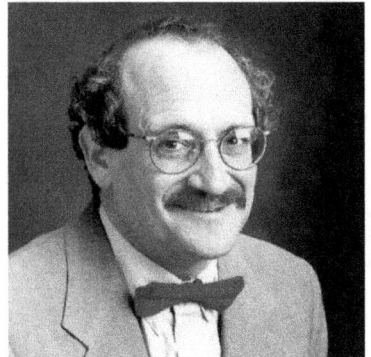

Dr. Jonathan Mann, who witnessed the tragedy that the AIDS epidemic brought to Africa in its early years, said that health is the right of all human beings. In 1986, as Director of the World Health Organization's Global Programme on AIDS (GPA), he led the global fight against AIDS. During his tenure, the World Health Organization allocated approximately one-third of its budget to AIDS-related programs.

However, due to internal problems, he had to leave the World Health Organization in 1990. AIDS programs slowed considerably for several years after he came out. Shortly after, he opened the François Xavier Bernard Center for Health and Human Rights at Harvard in Boston. He died in a plane crash in 1998. Had he worked at the World Health Organization for a few more years, the AIDS epidemic would have been under control much earlier.

Nathan Fain, Larry Kramer, and Larry Moss co-founded the Gay Men's Health Crisis (GMHC) in 1981. This is an organization that has made a significant contribution to the service of AIDS patients. The organization initiated a telephone hot line to provide moral support to AIDS patients. In July 1982, the first newsletter on AIDS was published. 50,000 copies were printed and distributed to patients, hospitals, clinics, and libraries. He ran a large program called 'Buddy' to meet the needs of AIDS victims. Programs are currently being organized for those who have been living with AIDS for a long time.

At Mount Sinai University School of Medicine in New York City, South African-born Dr. Joseph Adolph Sonnabend, an associate professor, treated his gay patients for opportunistic infections of AIDS and saved them for long periods of time, even before the availability of antiretroviral drugs. This demonstrated to the world that prophylactic treatment for numerous AIDS-related diseases could prolong the health of these patients even before the availability of antiretroviral drugs. Similarly, Dr. Sonnabend was instrumental in the creation of some of the largest AIDS patient service organizations and research organizations, such as the American Foundation for AIDS Research, the AIDS Community Research Initiative, the People with AIDS (PWA) Health Club, and the Buyers Club.

The Terrence Higgins Trust, named after the man who died of AIDS in Britain in the early days of the outbreak, has launched a large-scale consolation and awareness campaign for HIV patients. Feminist activists like Evelyn Hammonds, Linda Valle Rosa, and Kathy Cohen fought for the rights of HIV patients. In this way, after many humiliations, sufferings, and deaths, many people, including the victims of AIDS, have become the source of humanitarian-sympathetic struggles. Yet, despite some discrimination, AIDS victims enjoy almost equal status and respect in the wider society of wealthy countries. The situation in developing countries needs to be improved.

14. HIV and Tuberculosis

Tuberculosis, a global public health problem, is becoming more complex as people infected with HIV are more susceptible to TB.

Among the deadly opportunistic infections associated with AIDS are mainly viral, fungal, and parasitic diseases. Because tuberculosis is rare in the United States, whose AIDS medical guidelines are followed in a major part of the world, for a long time, they did not consider tuberculosis an opportunistic disease. In 1993, the CDC included tuberculosis as the most common life-threatening disease among HIV patients in developing and poor countries, along with recurrent bacterial pneumonia and invasive cervical cancer. However, tuberculosis accounts for the highest proportion of deaths among AIDS patients, at 27%.

Tuberculosis: The Ancient Scourge

Tuberculosis has been a scourge of humankind for thousands of years. It is estimated to have claimed about one billion lives throughout human history. On March 24, 1882, the German physician and pioneer of Microbiology, Robert Koch, demonstrated that the Acid-Fast Bacillus (now called *Mycobacterium tuberculosis*) was the causative agent of tuberculosis. It is estimated that one-quarter (25%) of the world's population is infected with TB. However, tuberculosis (TB) disease only manifests in an infected person when their immune system weakens due to several factors such as HIV, malnutrition, old age, diabetes, dialysis, smoking, chronic diseases, organ transplants, and treatment with steroids and cancer drugs.

Tuberculosis alone claims more lives than all other infectious diseases combined, making it the biggest global health problem. In 2022, tuberculosis affected 10.6 million people worldwide. More than 7.5 million people were diagnosed with TB in 2022 alone, and 1.3 million people died, of whom 187,000 were HIV patients. Malnutrition and diabetes, which weaken the immune system, typically trigger the emergence of this age-old disease that causes such havoc.

Tuberculosis in Developing vs. Developed Nations

Two hundred years ago, tuberculosis was prevalent almost all over the world. In the year 1632, out of 9,584 deaths in London, 1,797 were caused by tuberculosis (consumption). Since the 19th century, even before tuberculosis drugs were available, the disease prevalence has declined in industrialized countries in the Americas and Europe. It has been found that the disease can be effectively controlled by improving the quality of life rather than relying solely on medication.

In 1924, the BCG (Bacillus Calmette-Guérin) vaccine was introduced for tuberculosis. By the 1960s, the disease had almost disappeared in developed countries. It was thought that tuberculosis, which was prevalent in Africa, Asia, and South America, could be reduced by raising living standards. The 1950s saw the discovery and use of drugs for tuberculosis, beginning with streptomycin in 1944. However, due to economic backwardness, the disease is still affecting millions of people in developing countries. Poverty forces many people to live in rooms lacking proper ventilation and light, making it easy for tuberculosis patients to spread the bacterium to others.

Mycobacterium reach healthy people through the coughing, sneezing, talking, sputum expectoration of tuberculosis patients. Each patient can spread the bacteria to an average of 15 to 20 people. About 30 percent of the population into whom TB bacteria reached is infected. In those infected, about 95 percent of the immune system can effectively control the bacterium and prevent disease. This means that the bacteria are into dormancy. They have no symptoms. This is called latent TB. About 5% of those infected develop tuberculosis within a few weeks to two years. This is called primary progression. In the rest of the people due to the deficiency of nutrition and diabetes when the immune system becomes weak then becomes manifest disease tuberculosis. The symptoms include fever, cough, difficulty in breathing, fatigue, runny nose, headache, body aches, chills, and fatigue. The disease is called active TB. In tuberculosis which affects other organs than lungs symptoms depending on the organ. Lymph nodes are swollen in TB disease. TB Covering sack of heart (pericardium) leads to heart failure. Symptoms of intestinal TB include diarrhoea, while those of brain TB include headache, fits, and paralysis.

People with latent TB infection make up 85% of the population in a country with a high prevalence of infectious diseases, such as South Africa, compared to about 5% in a developed country, such as the United States. About 200 million people worldwide are infected with *Mycobacterium tuberculosis*. People with latent TB are susceptible to TB disease at any time in their lives - for any reason - when their immune system is weakened. Rare tuberculosis in the United States and other rich countries is exceedingly rare in those who were born and raised there. Tuberculosis occurs when the immunity of migrants from developing and poor countries is lowered for several reasons. TB of Reproductive system of women leads to infertility.

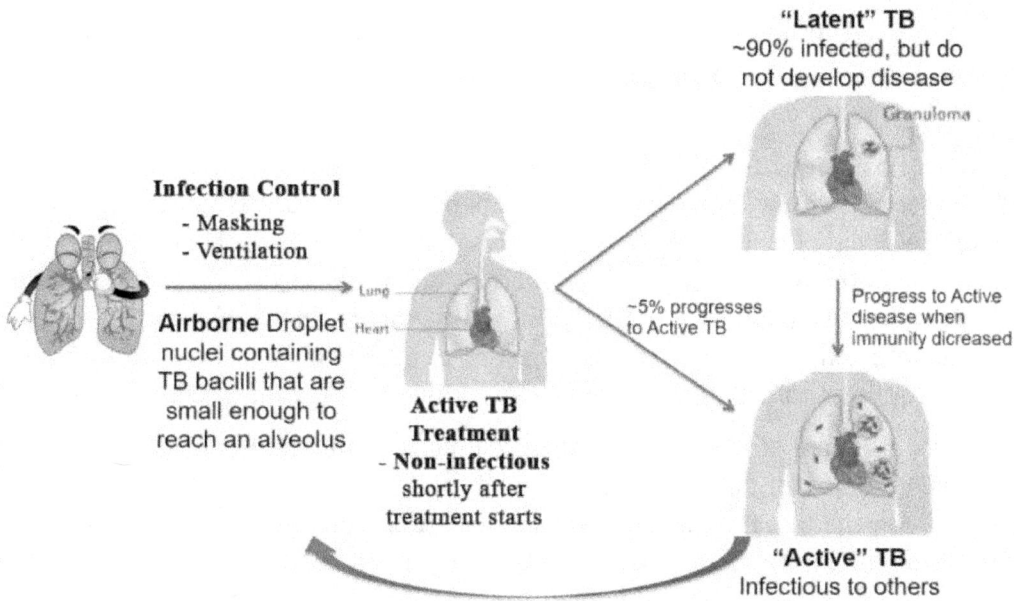

TB Transmission and Pathophysiology

Tuberculosis occurs mainly in America only in AIDS disease. About 70% of these immigrants come from outside the United States. This means that 70% of people who are infected with *Mycobacterium tuberculosis* as a child in their country of birth have a latent infection. Tuberculosis infection is a life-long infection. The virus is not transmitted from people with latent TB to others. It can only be transmitted from sick people to others.

Tuberculosis and HIV: A Deadly Combination

Primary progression, i.e., the chance of developing tuberculosis directly rather than as a latent infection after a tuberculosis infection, is only about 5% in the first two years of life in the general population. However, HIV patients have a higher lifetime risk of developing active tuberculosis through primary progression. The risk of developing active tuberculosis disease from latent TB infection is also too high in HIV patients.

Wearing a mask can help prevent the transmission of the infection to those around. Additionally, the room should be well-ventilated. Starting TB treatment reduces the probability of transmitting the bacterium to others, rendering patients non-infectious within a week or two.

Only pulmonary tuberculosis (lung tuberculosis) and laryngeal tuberculosis, among the many types of tuberculosis, can spread through the air. Tuberculosis can affect any part of the body, including the lungs, pleura (lung-sheath), lymph nodes, intestines, larynx, bones, spine, brain, skin, and reproductive system. In about 80 percent of people with the disease, tuberculosis affects the lungs. Tuberculosis that occurs outside of the lungs is called extrapulmonary TB.

Diagnosis, Treatment, and Prevention of Tuberculosis:

Diagnosis of latent TB: There are no symptoms in latent TB. The tuberculin skin test (Mantoux test) and interferon-gamma release assays (IGRAs) can diagnose latent TB.

Diagnosis of active TB: The disease can be diagnosed by performing certain tests on people with symptoms of tuberculosis, such as nucleic acid amplification tests (NAAT, e.g., GeneXpert) by Polymerase chain Reaction, chest X-ray, sputum acid-fast bacilli (AFB) test, urine lipoarabinomannan (LAM) test, TB culture, tuberculin skin test (Mantoux test). Additionally, depending on the organ suspected of being infected with tuberculosis in extra-pulmonary TB, CT scanning and a needle-sampling test called fine-needle aspiration cytology may also be required.

The principal drugs used in the treatment of tuberculosis are rifampicin, isoniazid, ethambutol, and pyrazinamide. Rifapentine replaces rifampicin in HIV patients. In the treatment of pulmonary tuberculosis and extrapulmonary tuberculosis, there is a difference not only in the medicines but also in the duration. Pulmonary TB is usually treated for 6 months, and extrapulmonary TB for 9–12 months.

Tuberculosis is a major health problem in many developing and poor countries, including India. Like AIDS, tuberculosis mainly affects the working class, and many families have lost their jobs and are in dire straits. HIV infection is on the rise all over the world.

Usually, the diagnosis of TB is often delayed. Patients repeatedly try several antibiotics for fever and cough without being aware of the potential for TB. In addition to this, patients often use fever pills and cough syrups from pharmacies without a doctor's prescription. This can lead to extensive disease and may lead to death if not treated on time. The diagnosis of extrapulmonary tuberculosis is more complicated and can take from 4 weeks to a few months. The characteristics of the tuberculous bacillus necessitate medication for a period ranging from six months to one and a half years. It is a long-term disease that progresses slowly. Some patients stop taking the drug on their own after 4–8 weeks once they feel better after starting treatment. This can cause the disease to worsen over time and become non-responsive (resistant) to the medications that were used earlier. This type of tuberculosis (multidrug-resistant TB, or MDR TB), which is not amenable to medication, is the most dangerous. In 2022, 40% of people infected with multi-drug-resistant TB will succumb to it. It can quickly infect others and require more expensive medications. However, the patient may still not survive. Tuberculosis patients should know that discontinuing treatment before the completion of the regimen is dangerous.

Since the 1980s, tuberculosis has re-emerged in industrialized countries with the emergence of HIV. Neglected tuberculosis research has rebounded in recent decades. This led to the development of the *Mycobacterium vaccae* vaccine for multidrug-resistant TB. The initial results are promising. A new drug called 'Rifapentine' was developed and introduced for the treatment of tuberculosis. Bedaquiline and Pretomanid were developed for the treatment of MDR-TB.

In 2018, the World Health Organization (WHO) declared tuberculosis a 'global emergency'. It provides technical and financial support by introducing innovative approaches to treating this disease. The treatment is being provided under the direct supervision of health workers. The government, NGOs, and doctors should regularly update their knowledge to identify the seriousness of tuberculosis and make people aware enough. The government should also implement anti-tuberculosis programs more vigorously. HIV infection, which greatly increases the chances of contracting tuberculosis, must be effectively curbed. Treating tuberculosis alone can increase the life expectancy of HIV-infected individuals by more than three years.

Global efforts to combat TB have saved seventy-five million lives since 2000.

Tuberculosis in HIV patients:

Tuberculosis in HIV patients is different from that in other patients. In non-HIV patients, TB slowly progresses. However, in people with HIV, tuberculosis, like bacterial pneumonia, may present acutely and severely. This complicates the diagnosis. That is, aggressive and rapid symptoms, rather than the slowly progressive symptoms present in tuberculosis. Slow convulsions, which become acute in a brief period of time, make the patient seriously ill. Tuberculosis can also lead to many complications if infected with HIV. Extrapulmonary tuberculosis (outside the lungs) in these patients is more common than in normal patients. With some HIV drugs, there are limitations (drug interactions) to the use of certain tuberculosis drugs in combination. In addition, relapses and recurrences are more common in HIV patients. All individuals with HIV should undergo TB testing. Additionally, all TB patients should be required to undergo HIV testing.

Although people with HIV can get infected with tuberculosis, those with HIV can become seriously ill and may end in death if not treated promptly. Although there is no cure for HIV, tuberculosis is curable. Timely diagnosis and treatment of the disease can help the patient recover.

The chances of developing tuberculosis in HIV patients are remarkably high. CD4+ lymphocytes play a vital role in immunity. When the number of these cells declines in HIV, they become victims of tuberculosis, which is prevalent in the world. Or if the tuberculosis bacilli are dormant in them, it may develop into a disease. Preventive therapy involves giving one or two TB drugs to HIV patients to prevent latent or active TB. In the same way that HIV Pre Exposure Prophylaxis (PrEP) is used as a 'treatment as prevention' with fewer drugs than regular treatment, suboptimal treatment is used for the prevention of tuberculosis from one month to nine months. All HIV patients are given preventive therapy without any testing for latent TB. HIV patients receive isoniazid for six to nine months as part of TB preventive therapy (TPT) for latent TB. There are also two-drug regimens that can be used for one to four months.*

The Global Burden of Tuberculosis:

HIV prevalence among tuberculosis (TB) patients continues to vary significantly by region and population. According to the latest data from the World Health Organization (WHO), globally, in 2021, an estimated 8.6% of the 10.6 million new TB cases were among people living with HIV. This translates to approximately 910,000 new TB cases among HIV-positive individuals worldwide. The burden remains disproportionately higher in sub-Saharan Africa, where the overall estimate of HIV prevalence among TB patients was 34% in 2021. Within this region, some countries face a particularly severe dual epidemic, with HIV prevalence among TB patients reaching as high as 60% in certain parts of South Africa. In contrast, other regions like Southeast Asia and the Western Pacific have relatively lower HIV prevalence among TB patients, at 4.1% and 3.5%, respectively, in 2021. These latest figures reiterate the urgent need for continued and intensified efforts to integrate HIV and TB services, particularly in regions grappling with a high dual burden of these deadly diseases.

India's Struggle with Tuberculosis and HIV:

According to the World Health Organization (WHO), India has the highest number of TB patients in the world. In 2020, 26% of the world's TB patients were in India. In 2021, a total of 1,933,381 people were diagnosed with tuberculosis in India. Of these, 50,000 are HIV-positive. 3.4% of people with tuberculosis have HIV. The rise in cases speaks to the seriousness of the TB problem in India. One in four AIDS-related deaths in India, or 25 percent, is due to tuberculosis. In 2021, 210 new cases of TB were reported annually per 100,000 people in India. In the United States, only three out of every 100,000 people suffer from tuberculosis. In South Africa, where tuberculosis is the most common, it affects about 1,000 people per 100,000 people.

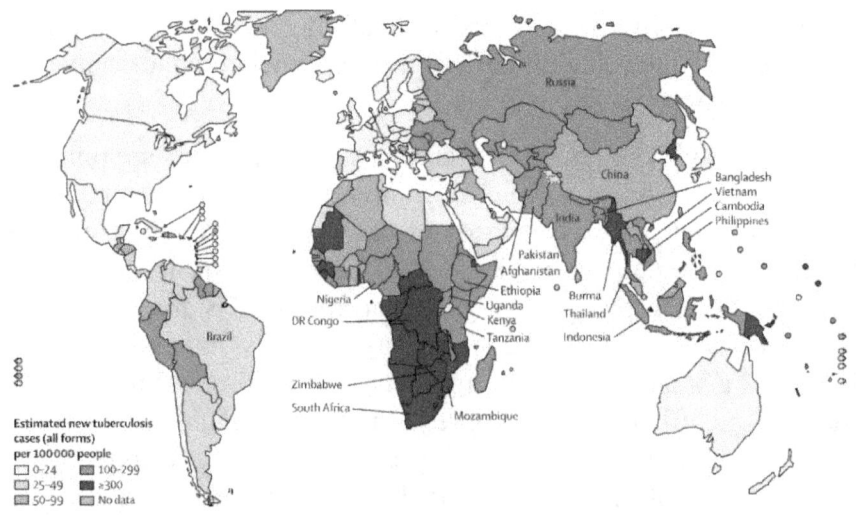

Prevalence of Tuberculosis in various countries

India, which is currently the number one country in the world in terms of population, is embarrassingly number one with the highest number of TB patients in the world. We are in the third position in terms of HIV patients. However, it is a matter of some relief that the health sector is doing somewhat better, and India is in the second position in terms of TB deaths.

* The author is of the view that preventive therapy is not required in infectious diseases when the time of exposure is indefinite, and the risk of developing disease in HIV is independent of the CD4+ lymphocyte count. Tuberculosis manifests at any stage of HIV disease, regardless of the CD4+ count. In the early years of AIDS, all patients in the United States were given up to twenty pills each day to prevent them from contracting several opportunistic diseases, and the same was practiced in many developed countries. This rule is not in force at present. The author also does not believe there is a need for such preventive therapy for tuberculosis.

15. Tuberculin response to assess AIDS severity in HIV- TB patients

Dr. Yanamadala concluded that the TB 'diagnostic' test can be used to assess the severity of AIDS in HIV-TB patients and that the test has a limited role in diagnosing TB in them.

The Challenge of Diagnosing TB in HIV Patients:

My research is on what the response of the tuberculin (Mantoux) test indicates in HIV patients infected with tuberculosis. Most HIV patients are affected with tuberculosis. About 70 to 80 percent of HIV patients in developing/poor countries are affected with tuberculosis. About 30% of people with AIDS die from tuberculosis.

As part of the tuberculosis diagnosis in children (adults), a skin injection test (Mantoux) is performed. Tuberculin (Purified Protein Derivative, or PPD) is injected into the skin of the forearm. Tuberculosis is diagnosed based on the diameter of the induration on the skin between 48 and 72 hours. This rash is caused by a reaction of the patient's immune system. If they have an induration larger than 10 millimetres, they are diagnosed with tuberculosis.

However, experts suggest that in HIV patients, tuberculosis can be diagnosed if the induration is more than 5 millimetres. CD4+ lymphocytes (T-helper cells) play a key role in the induration response. HIV infects and destroys CD4+ lymphocytes in HIV patients. This leads to a blunted test response. Therefore, the induration limit to diagnose TB has been reduced to 5 mm instead of 10 mm in the general population. But I had a different idea.

Implications of Tuberculin Response in Assessing AIDS Severity:

Since the response is based on cell-mediated immunity, which depends on the number (activity) of CD4+ cells, and in HIV, these cell numbers are declining with severity, what is the relevance of putting a limit of 5 millimetres?

However, not much research has been done on the relationship between the tuberculin response in HIV-TB and the severity of AIDS. I conducted research on the patients in the hospital to look at the issue in depth.

Research Methodology:

In my research, 10 units of tuberculin antigen (PPD) was injected into each of 107 HIV patients who were diagnosed with tuberculosis with symptoms, sputum testing, and chest X-rays. I also performed the same test on 100 other HIV-negative tuberculosis patients. On the third day, I checked the injection site. I also checked the physical condition of all the patients. The HIV patients who participated in the study were not on antiretroviral drugs.

Research Findings and Implications:

Surprisingly, in HIV-TB patients, the size of induration ranged from no blistering at all (anergy) to 26 millimetres. This indicates that the Mantoux test plays a limited role in diagnosing tuberculosis in HIV patients.

Of the 107 HIV-TB patients, 33 had an induration greater than 10 mm. Thirty of them were slightly underweight. Within six weeks in the hospital, 33 patients (100%) had improved their health with treatment. They were advised to continue their medicines and discharged from the hospital.

Of the 26 HIV-TB patients who showed a response of 5 to 10 millimetres of induration, 20 (79 percent) recovered after more than a month and a half in the hospital. Six people had died (21%). All 26 patients were emaciated.

In 48 patients, the response to the Mantoux test was 5mm or less or no response at all. Of these, 42 were severely wasted. The remaining six (12.5 percent) with a normal build were discharged after prolonged hospitalization. Of the remaining, 30 (62.5%) died, while the remaining 12 (25%) left the hospital without informing the doctors.

Out of 100 non-HIV infected tuberculosis patients, only three (3%) died.

What does the research uncover?

The study found that people infected with HIV in developing countries, such as India, were more likely to develop tuberculosis. Regardless of the stage of the disease, they become ill with tuberculosis without much loss of immunity, as evidenced by 26 mm of induration.

Patients who show an induration of more than 10 millimetres in the tuberculin test are in the early stages of HIV. They all recovered.

Those with an induration of 6 to 10 millimetres showed a slightly higher severity of the disease. They were all wasted.

The disease appears to be highly advanced in HIV-TB patients who do not respond or respond less than 5 mm to the tuberculin test.

In developing countries like India, it has been shown to be useful in prescribing appropriate treatment to the patient by assessing the severity of HIV at a very low cost, considering our limitations. Then I examined the relationship between the diameter of induration and patient recovery. Patients showing less than 5 mm of induration had the worst outcome; most of them died.

The majority of those who showed induration between 6 and 10 millimetres needed prolonged hospital treatment and recovered, but some of them died.

All patients with more than 10 millimetres of induration recovered quickly.

In HIV patients with tuberculosis, there is a relationship between the response to the Mantoux test and the severity of their disease. The relationship is consistent, with uniform results across separate groups. I proposed using the Mantoux test in HIV patients with TB as a prognostic marker to gauge the severity of HIV. I proposed devising a scale-like approach by conducting research with a large number of patients and comparing the results with the CD4+ count. This implies that we could replace more expensive tests to assess the severity of a new disease with a low-tech, widely available, and cheap diagnostic test.

A Cost-Effective Solution for Assessing AIDS Severity:

Dr. Yanamadala says that the solution to our health problems should be in the form of inexpensive methods, keeping in mind the limited resources available to us. In developing countries, estimating the severity of AIDS is unaffordable. The CD4+ lymphocyte count and viral load tests currently used to assess the severity of AIDS are about four thousand rupees (50 USD) expensive. These tests are only available in urban areas. In such a situation, there is a need to find inexpensive ways to determine the severity of AIDS in poor countries, a disease that mostly affects poor people. In July 2000, I presented this scientific abstract (Prognostic Implications of Tuberculin Responsiveness in HIV Infection with Tuberculosis, WePeC4410) to the 13th World AIDS Conference in Durban, South Africa.

Recognition and Impact of the Research:

The 13th International AIDS Conference was the first international AIDS conference held in a developing country. The conference approved and published five thousand abstracts from all over the world. After the conference, the renowned medical website Medscape published the key points of the conference with 25 outstanding research abstracts.

Dr. Yanamadala's Scientific Abstract in XIII International AIDS Conference

HIV-AIDS

My research was one of those outstanding. AIDS-related tuberculosis is the subject of 10 out of 25 abstracts. Eight of them were from Africa, one from the USA, and one was mine. This article has also been published in some journals.

Dr. Yanamadala's Abstract in Medscape

The study was conducted between 1997 and 2000 at Rangaraya Medical College, Kakinada, Andhra Pradesh. The then Professor of Tuberculosis, Dr. Sunnam Satya Sri, and colleagues from the Department of Microbiology helped.

Scan the QR code for the article of 25 great research papers selected by Medscape.

16. HIV and Pregnancy

Because of the many personal, social, and health problems associated with HIV and infected pregnancy, all factors must be considered before conceiving.

About 85% of HIV-infected women are of childbearing age. In almost all societies, it is natural for couples to have children. HIV is primarily transmitted through sex. Pregnancy is an extension of sexual life. For people living with HIV infection before pregnancy, there are many things to keep in mind if they want to have a baby.

Understanding Mother-to-Child Transmission:

Various studies in the early years of the AIDS epidemic have shown that the virus infected 15 to 30 out of 100 children born to HIV-positive mothers.

Not all infants born to HIV-positive mothers contract HIV; some do. For instance, take two babies. Two children can be healthy; in other instances, only one of them can be infected with HIV, or both can be infected with HIV. It is a myth that a mother gives birth to a child by sharing her blood. There is no blood supply to the foetus from the mother. A baby in the womb produces blood for her own body. The placenta only transmits essential nutrients such as amino acids, glucose, fats, small proteins, and oxygen from mother to child. Because of this, the chances of passing HIV from mother to foetus are low.

Factors Influencing Transmission Risk:

If the labour (delivery) of a woman with HIV is prolonged, the chances of the child contracting HIV increase. If the labour is difficult and there are traumatic injuries, such as bleeding in the birth tract or any diseases in the genitals of the mother, the baby getting infected is more likely. Similarly, the risk of transmitting the virus to the baby is higher in people with an advanced stage of the disease due to the high viral load. The viral load is usually high in the early months of HIV infection and in the advanced stages of the disease. Pregnancy in these cases is not advisable because of the risk of infection for the unborn baby. If a woman is affected by infectious diseases such as typhoid, pneumonia, tuberculosis and herpes during pregnancy, the viral load increases significantly for a few weeks. In such cases, the risk of infection for the baby increases.

One major risk factor is chorioamnionitis, which is an infection of the membranes surrounding the baby in the womb. This disrupts the placenta's protective barrier and allows HIV-infected cells to enter the amniotic fluid surrounding the baby. Having other sexually transmitted infections (STIs) like syphilis, gonorrhoea, or chlamydia has also been linked to higher rates of HIV transmission from mother to child.

During pregnancy, sometimes there is a risk of bleeding into the uterus. This is more likely to happen during delivery. If the baby is exposed to the mother's blood or blood-stained womb fluid for a prolonged period of time, the chances of passing HIV to the baby increase. The same thing happens in the podalic version. Attempts by obstetricians to change the position of the baby (such as a podalic version), which is performed to change the baby's head position for smooth delivery, can increase the chances of the baby contracting HIV. Amniocentesis, a method of testing the water of the womb to detect genetic or other defects in the foetus, also increases the chances of the baby being infected with HIV.

Unprotected sexual intercourse (without a condom) during pregnancy itself is thought to be associated with an increased risk of mother-to-child transmission of HIV. Multiple pregnancies, like twins or triplets, also increase the likelihood of a baby getting HIV.

The PACTG 076 Study & Nevirapine

Before the introduction of three-drug combination therapy, the United States conducted the PACTG 076 (Paediatric AIDS Clinical Trials Group 076) study in 1994, which marked a significant milestone in the pregnancy of HIV-infected women. One group of 556 pregnant women received 100 mg tablets of Zidovudine five times a day starting from the second trimester of pregnancy, or 14 weeks. They received Zidovudine in the form of saline during delivery. The newborn was also given Zidovudine syrup for six weeks. In the other group, neither the mother nor the child were given any HIV drugs. The children in both groups were tested for HIV at specific intervals over an 18-month period.

About 8.3 percent (about 8 per 100) of the children who were given Zidovudine were found to be infected with HIV. 25.5 percent (one quarter) of children born to women who did not use any medication were diagnosed with HIV infection. The study showed that two-thirds (67.5%) of children were protected against HIV infection with the use of Zidovudine. Babies born in the Zidovudine group were not breastfed. In this way, HIV infection is prevented during infancy.

A study of affordable Nevirapine in South Africa, Zimbabwe, Uganda, and Tanzania, published in the Lancet, is a small relief for countries where no retro-viral drugs are available. To reduce mother-to-child transmission of HIV, a pregnant woman is given one dose of Nevirapine 200 mg immediately after the onset of labour pains, and the newborn is given Nevirapine syrup for six weeks. Stopped sneezing. Giving Nevirapine to mothers and children reduced HIV infection by half compared to those who did not receive any medication. However, there were concerns over this single-drug therapy; even at a single dose, HIV developed resistance to the drug.

The PROMISE Trial and Current Practices:

In 2017, the New England Journal of Medicine announced the PROMISE trial, which discussed the results of various antiretroviral drugs in 3529 HIV-positive pregnant women. The study was conducted in India, South Africa, Malawi, Tanzania, Zimbabwe, Zambia, and Uganda. They all have a CD4+ lymphocyte count above 350. Until then, only Zidovudine (PACTG 076) was used in the second trimester for pregnant women. The pregnant women were divided into three groups. Those in the first group were given only Zidovudine. The mother was given Nevirapine during childbirth. The child was given a tenofovir-Emtricitabine combination for four weeks. In the second group, pregnant women were given Zidovudine-Lamivudine-Ritonavir-boosted Lopinavir. The child was given the same medicine for four weeks. Pregnant women in the third group were given tenofovir, Emtricitabine, and Ritonavir-boosted Lopinavir. The child was given the same medicine for four weeks.

In the first group of pregnant women given the same drug, 1.8 percent (almost two out of 100) of the children were infected. In the Zidovudine-Lamivudine-Ritonavir boosted Lopinavir group, 0.5% (i.e., 1 in 200) of the children were infected with HIV. In the third group, 0.6 percent (about 1 in 200) of the children were infected with HIV from their mother.

Regardless of her CD4+ count, administering a regular standard three-drug combination of HIV medication to an HIV-infected woman from the second trimester of pregnancy significantly reduced the risk of HIV transmission to the unborn child. That is why pregnant women are now being given regular, standard HIV treatment.

Modern Approaches in Prevention of Transmission:

A polymerase chain reaction (PCR) test is done to determine whether a baby born to an HIV-infected woman is not infected with the virus. ELISA and Western blot tests are tests that detect antibodies but are not chosen because antibodies can be passed from mother to child even if the virus is not transmitted. PCR tests detect the virus. Antibodies passed from mother to child disappear after 18 months. After 18 months, the result can be confirmed by antibody tests, namely ELISA or Western Blot.

The earlier practice was to have a caesarean operation (also known as an elective caesarean section) before the onset of labour (delivery) pains, a week or two before expected delivery, to reduce the chances of HIV transmission. It is now believed that the surgery is not necessary just to prevent the child from contracting HIV. Suspension of breastfeeding is also important to prevent the baby from getting HIV.

Giving birth prematurely (before 37 weeks of pregnancy) increases the risk of a mother passing HIV to her baby. This is because premature babies have weaker immune systems, and tender, vulnerable skin is more likely to be exposed to HIV-infected fluids during delivery. Preterm births are often associated with infections of the foetal membranes that can disrupt the placenta's protective barrier. Premature deliveries also tend to involve higher viral loads in the mother, further raising the transmission risk.

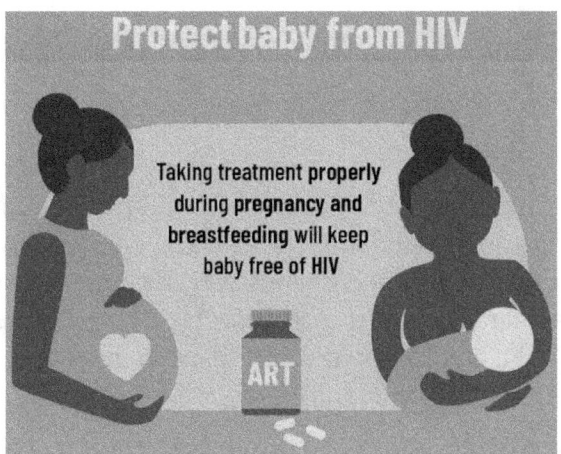

If a child born to an HIV-infected woman is not infected with HIV at birth, there is a minimal chance that the child will later be infected through lactation. In fact, in developing countries, the percentage of children who die from HIV acquired through breastfeeding is lower than the percentage of children who die from other infections and malnutrition that formula milk may bring. A lot of care needs to be taken when it comes to feeding other than the breastmilk of the mother. Children are often at risk of diarrhoea, respiratory diseases, and malnutrition if caregivers do not take precautions, such as cleaning their hands, and the water content in the baby's feed increases. We must exercise caution in this regard. It is good that only those who can afford the expenses in case of any disease should opt for formula milk. Otherwise, it is better to breastfeed an HIV-positive mother.

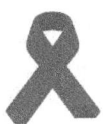

17. Living with HIV

Antiretroviral drugs, nutrition, hygiene, and avoiding infections help HIV-infected people live longer and healthier.

Infectious diseases are rare in developed countries due to their high standards of living. Clean water, balanced nutrition, and personal-environmental hygiene prevent the growth of pathogens there. However, for people in developing and poor countries, living standards are low due to a lack of basic resources. Therefore, pathogens present in the environment cause diseases in people with low immunity. The immune system needs to be healthy to function optimally.

Protect Immune System by Avoiding other Infections:

People infected with the HIV that causes AIDS can live normally for many years after infection. However, by taking some precautions, they can live longer. An HIV-infected person's immune system is weakened, making them more susceptible to various infections. By avoiding such diseases, their quality of life improves, and their lifespan increases. Each time an HIV person contracts other pathogens, it insults their immune system. During an infection, the virus replicates in dormant cells, causing a decline in the number of CD4+ cells. CD4+ lymphocytes do not replenish as quickly as they are reduced. Therefore, there is an increasing susceptibility to various infectious diseases. Hence, HIV patients should be vigilant about not contracting any disease, making it a part of their lifestyle. Before CD4+ lymphocytes decline significantly, patients are vulnerable to milder forms of infectious diseases.

Usually, people infected with HIV are more likely to contract various serious infections 6 to 12 years after being infected, as their CD4+ lymphocyte count reaches a low. Since there is always a risk of contracting severe diseases, HIV-infected people should protect themselves from infection from the very beginning. People with HIV do not have to stop working. They can continue in their professions, jobs, and businesses as long as they have the energy to work.

Healthy Habits for HIV: Diet, Hygiene, and Rest:

A healthy diet will boost the immune system. A well-balanced diet consisting of milk, eggs, meat, pulses, beans, and fruits helps in the proper functioning of white blood cells, which play a key role in immunity. Although diets in developing countries are full, there is not enough protein to meet the body's nutritional needs and maintain health. As a result, immune cells are unable to function optimally, and antibodies are not produced adequately. This often leads to the development of diseases.

People with HIV should stay away from people with colds, typhoid, tuberculosis, and various fevers as much as possible. People infected with HIV should avoid those who have a fever and cough. Tuberculosis is the number one killer of HIV-infected people worldwide. If any family member is suffering from TB, it is better to stay elsewhere until the disease improves. Along with taking precautions against various diseases, one can reduce the stress on the immune system as much as possible by taking appropriate treatment in time for any illness. HIV patients can live a long life.

Preventing Infections Through Hygiene:

The most important aspect of personal hygiene is that the microbes causing various diseases usually enter the body through the air, contaminated food, drinks, and hands. Therefore, maintaining hygiene in things like food and drinking water is crucial.

Correct way of using a sanitary latrine

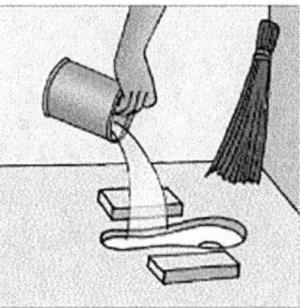

First pour a little water into the pan to make it wet

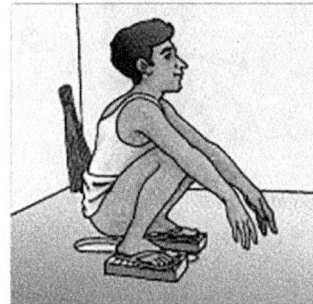

Sit across the pan and defecate

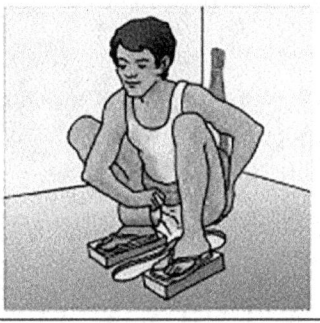

After defecating, clean yourself with water

Pour water into the pan to flush down the excreta

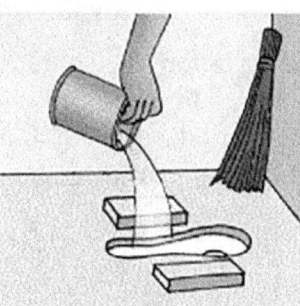

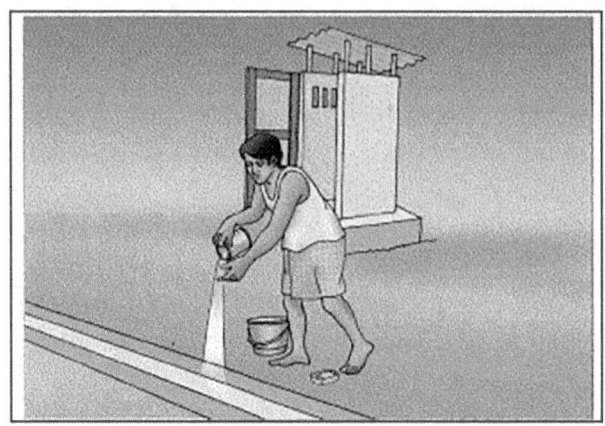
After urinating and passing stools, always wash hands with soap and water.

Washing hands thoroughly with soap and water before eating any food is a must. Street food with roaming insects like flies should not be eaten in such conditions. Bacteria that do not cause much harm to healthy people can cause diseases in those infected with HIV. Drink only filtered or boiled water. Carry drinking water and food from home during travel. Wash hands with soap/ash thoroughly after defecation and urination.

Managing Stress and Anxiety in HIV:

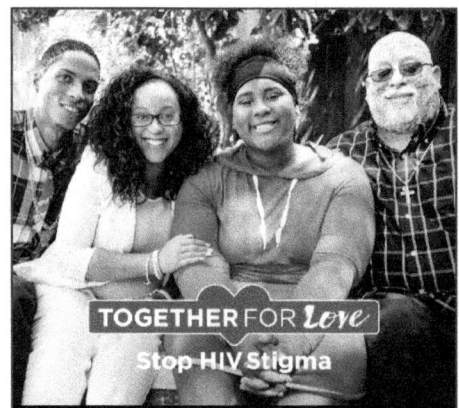

It is greatly beneficial for them to have peace of mind. An HIV-infected person's health can quickly deteriorate due to stress and anxiety. Therefore, they can be encouraged by spending enough time on activities of their choice, such as book reading and cultural and recreational activities. Discussing bothersome issues and problems with close, trusted friends and family members brings some comfort.

Adequate sleep is essential for the immune system to function optimally. People say they suffer from a cold after travel trips for some days due to a change of water. In fact, a lack of sleep during travel can weaken the immune system and make it easier to catch a cold.

Avoid Harmful Substances to Protect Immune System:

Consumption of alcohol, tobacco, and tobacco products often leads to respiratory infections. Therefore, it is not advisable for HIV-infected people to smoke. Drugs belonging to the class of corticosteroids, such as dexamethasone, reduce immunity. Therefore, no medicine should be taken without a doctor's prescription.

HIV and Life Expectancy: Treatment and Lifestyle

With better access to HIV treatment, life expectancy has increased significantly in countries like the United States and Europe. In the US, the average life expectancy for people without HIV is 80 years, while those with HIV live close to 74 years. However, in poor and developing countries, the life expectancy of HIV patients is still short due to the late availability of HIV drugs, the presence of many diseases, and the lack of an adequate standard of living. With a healthy lifestyle, one can live almost the same length of time as the rest of the population in these countries.

It is sad that some people end their lives by committing suicide due to fear of social stigma regarding HIV infection. All people should support and respect HIV patients, just like everyone else. Ostracizing them is a blot on humanity. Even those who cannot afford anti-HIV drugs can live some more years with effective treatment of infectious diseases such as tuberculosis and a healthy lifestyle. HIV/AIDS is like many other chronic diseases. It does not need to be depressed. The advice of doctors is helpful for those suffering from this disease to live with optimism.

18. HIV Cure Research

Although complex and expensive treatments for other diseases in HIV patients can cure HIV, they are not feasible for everyone. Currently, research is moving in a different direction.

Everything in nature is interdependent, including humans and other animals. Only a small number of microbes that infect humans cause disease. Retroposons, which make up about six percent of human DNA, are genes from a variety of viruses with which humans have come into contact for millions of years. They became part of human DNA. The DNA of an HIV-infected person has added nine genes.

The Challenge of HIV Eradication:

HIV infection in these cells can occur through two main pathways:
I. Productive (or lytic) infection: In this case, the HIV genome integrates into the host cell's DNA, and the cell becomes a factory for producing new viral particles. This process ultimately leads to the lysis (rupturing) and death of the infected cell, releasing new virions that can go on to infect other cells.

In productive infection, the infected cells will be positive for proviral DNA (integrated viral genome), HIV RNA (viral genetic material being transcribed), and HIV proteins (viral proteins being produced).

The continuous depletion of CD4++ T cells is a hallmark of HIV infection and the progression to AIDS. As these cells are critical for coordinating the immune response, their loss leads to a weakened immune system and increased susceptibility to various opportunistic infections and certain cancers.

II. Latent (or non-productive) infection: In this case, the HIV genome integrates into the host cell's DNA, but the virus remains dormant and does not actively produce new virions. These cells are known as viral reservoirs and can harbour the virus for lengthy periods without being detected or eliminated by the immune system.

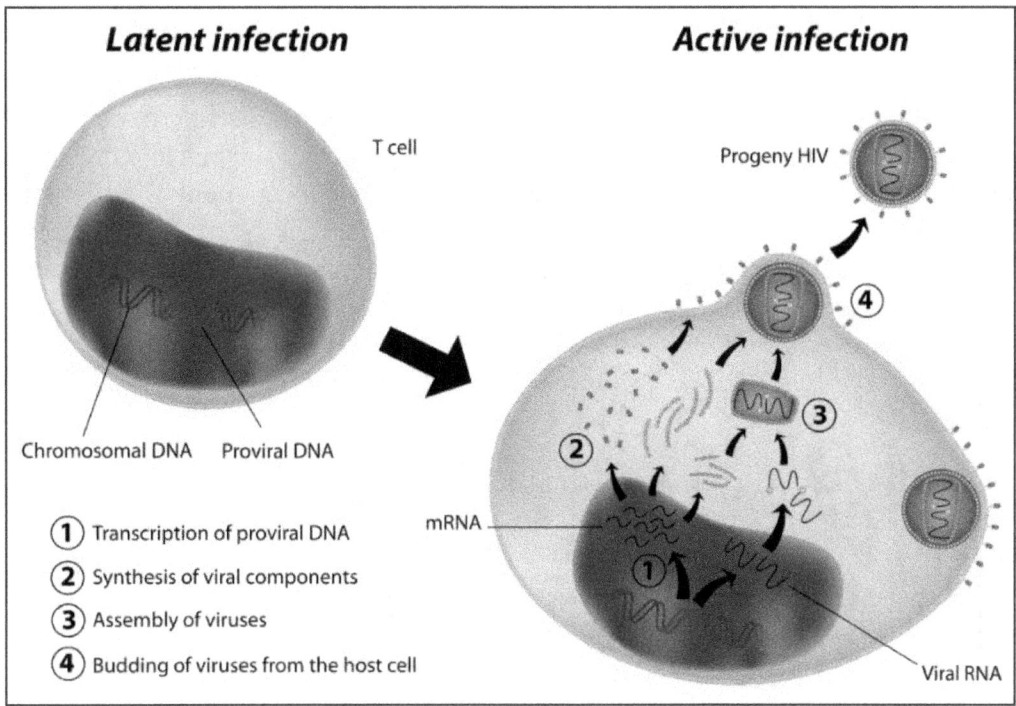

Another type is a latent infection. It is called a reservoir, and they do not replicate and stay quiescent. In latent cells, only proviral DNA is positive, whereas RNA is negative. The HIV protein is also negative. As a result, the body's immune system does not recognize it, and the cell remains alive for a long time. It is possible for one type of cell to become another. Currently available anti-HIV drugs can control only the productive infection. However, latent cells do not show any signs of the virus. This is the real obstacle to the complete eradication of HIV.

HIV cures are of two types. One is a sterilizing cure; the second is a functional cure. If HIV is eliminated without any signs, it is called a sterilizing cure. So far, six patients have been completely cured of HIV. All of them were cured of the virus through stem cell therapy given for another life-threatening disease. Gene therapy may also achieve this in the future.

Stem Cell Therapy: A Potential Cure with Limitations

Professor Stein O'Brien, an HIV, and genetics researcher at Harvard University, has observed that some people who have been exposed to HIV for a long time do not become infected with the virus. The reason for this is that HIV infection requires a CD4+ protein as well as a co-receptor (CCR5), and people with this genetic mutation that renders CCR5-deficient are not infected with HIV.

Stem cells from a donor with a homozygous CCR5 Δ32 mutation, which does not make the CCR5 coreceptor in the body, can be given to an HIV patient and rid them of the virus. About one percent of Europeans (Caucasians) carry the CCR5 Δ32 mutation. However, finding suitable donors with this rare genetic mutation is extremely challenging, making this treatment accessible to only an exceedingly small number of individuals.

Timothy Ray Brown, popularly known as the Berlin Patient, was an AIDS patient. In 2006, he was treated with a stem cell transplant or bone marrow transplant by Dr. Gero Hutter of Heidelberg University as part of treatment for his acute myeloid leukaemia, a blood cancer. In 2009, researchers discovered that Timothy Ray Brown did not have HIV. Timothy Ray Brown achieved the first-ever HIV cure. He died of cancer in September 2020.

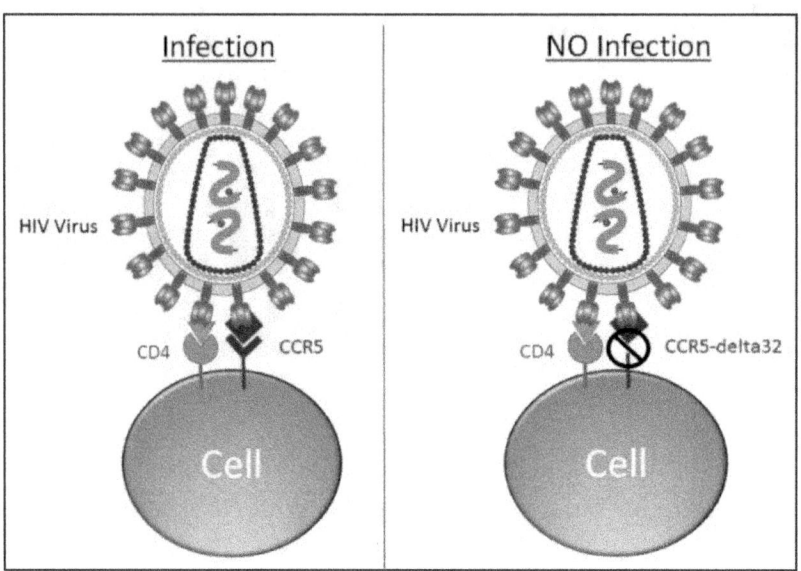

The 'New York Patient' was the first woman to be cured of HIV. She became HIV-free in February 2022.

In 2018, another man from Switzerland developed complications after a stem cell transplant and was later cured of HIV. The doctors discovered a new development involving him, known as the Geneva Patient. Previously, it was believed that the only way to eradicate HIV was through the transplantation of stem cells from a homozygous individual lacking CCR5 in both parents. The man who donated stem cells to this Geneva patient had only one missing gene from one parent. This is called heterozygosity. Stem cells collected from heterozygous donors are also known to be helpful in getting rid of HIV.

HIV Cure strategies that seem promising

Targeting Infected Cell
- Very early ART
- Latency reversal
- Latency silencing
- Gene editing

Activating Immune System
- bNAbs
- T cell vaccines
- Immunomodulation
- CAR T cells

    It is not a treatment that can be provided to all patients under normal conditions. We are all mostly familiar with kidney transplantation and liver transplantation. Many types of immunosuppressant medicines should be used so that the recipient's body does not reject the organs introduced from another person's body. Therefore, the transplanted person is susceptible to various infections throughout life. Such a problem occurs more often when the bone marrow / stem cells that produce immune cells are to be transplanted. Therefore, potent immunosuppression is required. That is, getting rid of HIV through the treatment of stem cells / bone marrow transplants in this way means falling from the fry pan into the fireplace. This is actively seeking problems. It is estimated that about one percent of Caucasians are CCR5-negative. The donor and the patient who needs stem cell therapy must be genetically compatible. Stem cell therapy is much more difficult and problematic than any other transplant. Sometimes a severe type of rejection reaction called graft versus host disease (GvHD) is seen. It is a very complex process. Stem cell therapy has been counterproductive for many patients.

    Stem cell therapy (such a large number of donors without the CCR5 protein is unlikely to be available!) mandates immunosuppressant treatment. It is to be taken throughout life post-treatment, which is even more complicated and more expensive than HIV treatment! People who undergo this treatment are more susceptible to infections. It is impossible for all HIV patients to be cured of HIV in the same way that they were accidentally cured of HIV as part of the treatment for leukaemia or cancer. Currently, available HIV treatment is remarkably effective and not very expensive, although HIV cannot be completely eradicated.

Gene Therapy: Editing the Path to a Cure

With gene therapy, attempts are made to create a similar CCR5-negative condition. CRISPR/Cas9 ('Clustered Regularly Interspaced Short Palindromic Repeats' / Cas9 Enzyme) gene scissors are used to inhibit CCR5, the CD4+ co-receptor. This involves cutting and deleting the target HIV gene that is integrated into the human DNA.

With this kind of gene and cell therapy, scientists have already been able to give a complete cure to about 30 genetic diseases, and some serious birth defects due to 'one gene defect' have been completely cured by inserting the relevant gene into the patient's DNA. Leber congenital amaurosis (LCA), a rare form of spinal muscular atrophy, beta thalassemia, sickle cell anaemia, haemophilia, cystic fibrosis, etc. Patients who previously had no life with these diseases are now able to live a full, normal life.

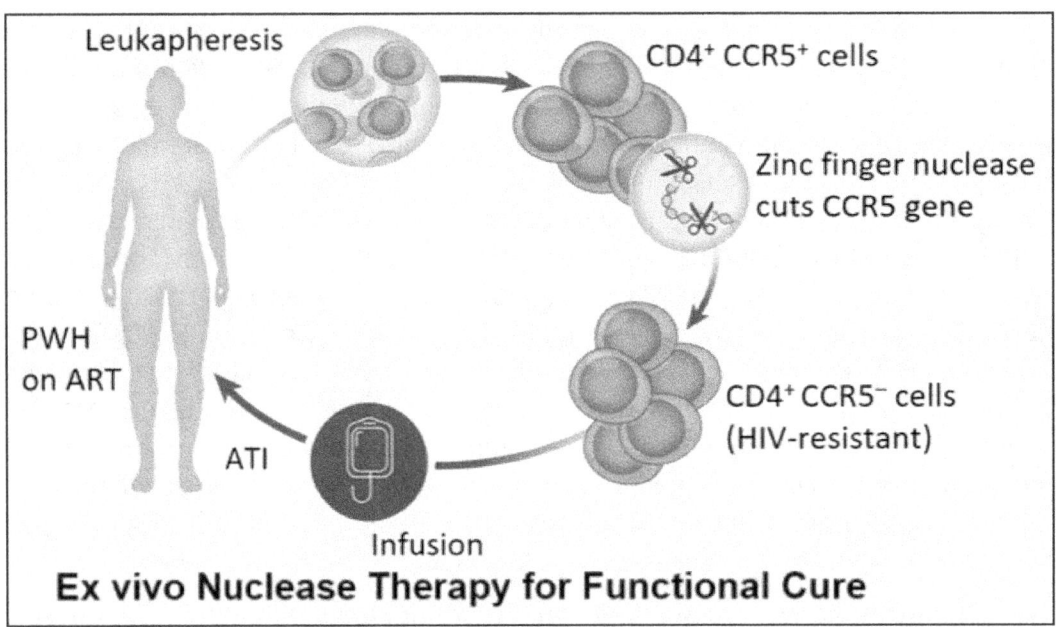

Nuclease-based gene therapy holds significant promise for achieving a functional cure for HIV infection. This approach involves using engineered nucleases, such as zinc finger nucleases (ZFNs), transcription activator-like effector nucleases (TALENs), or the CRISPR/Cas9 system, to specifically target and disrupt the CCR5 gene, which encodes a co-receptor essential for HIV entry into CD4++ T cells.

Ex vivo gene editing:

The patient's CD4++ T cells, or hematopoietic stem/progenitor cells (HSPCs), are collected from their blood or bone marrow.

The cells are exposed to the nuclease system (ZFNs, TALENs, or CRISPR/Cas9) designed to target and disrupt the CCR5 gene.

The gene-edited cells are then expanded in vitro (laboratory) and reinfused back into the patient.

There is also another approach: in vivo gene editing. The nuclease system is delivered directly to the patient's body, typically through viral vectors or nanoparticle delivery systems.

This approach has shown promising results in animal studies and early-stage clinical trials. However, several challenges need to be addressed.

While promising, CRISPR technology for HIV treatment is still in its preliminary stages, with ongoing research and clinical trials exploring its safety and efficacy.

Functional Cure: Controlling HIV Without Eradication

Functional cure means the virus genes remain in some cells of the body but are not able to replicate and grow. Antibodies introduced from outside destroy the latent cells that have HIV genes and are not replicating. It is believed that HIV can be eradicated by making such latent cells productive and destroying them with antiretrovirals and the body's immune system. Research is also underway for latency-reversing agents to eliminate latent cells. This is called the shock-and-kill method.

Latent cells produce a protein called BCL2. Some types of cancer cells also produce this BCL2. The antibody Venetoclax, which treats chronic lymphocytic leukaemia, destroys these BCL2 cells. Research is being carried out to eliminate latent or reservoir cells infected with HIV using them. Similarly, antibodies produced against PD1 and CTL A4 molecules were also found to be useful in reducing HIV reservoir loads. It is called block and lock. Other research avenues for a functional cure include therapeutic vaccines aimed at boosting the immune system's ability to control HIV and broadly neutralizing antibodies capable of targeting a wide range of HIV strains.

Elite Controllers & Long-Term Non-Progressors: Clues to a Cure

Scientists have found that a ridiculously small number of patients infected with HIV are able to live a healthy life without medication for a long time. They are known as long-time non-progressors (LTNP) and elite controllers (EC). Researchers are actively studying these individuals to understand the mechanisms behind their HIV control, hoping to translate these findings into new treatment strategies for all people living with HIV.

The Importance of Early Intervention:

In 2020, Lorraine Willenberg, a patient in San Francisco who had been HIV positive for 25 years, stopped taking HIV drugs three years earlier, but the virus had not rebounded. We all know that some types of cancer are curable after treatment. This is called remission.

In the Visconti study announced by French doctors in 2022, six men and four women started treatment less than three months after being infected with HIV. They all received HIV treatment for at least a year. Seven of them had a nearly undetectable HIV viral load for more than 10 years, despite stopping treatment. One of them had an undetectable viral load for 17 years. Three of them were given antiretroviral therapy due to their high viral load. After reviewing several such studies, it is estimated that if treatment is started in the early days of HIV infection, 5% of patients will not develop the virus until later in life, even without HIV treatment.

However, early detection of infection with HIV, known as acute HIV infection, is rare in developing countries. This underscores the critical importance of early HIV diagnosis and immediate access to antiretroviral therapy, especially in developing countries where healthcare resources may be limited.

19. The Promise and challenge of an AIDS Vaccine

The high genetic diversity and mutations unique to HIV make it difficult to develop a vaccine for the disease.

Vaccines introduced to prevent infections in human history have literally changed the face of the world. Scientists were able to develop vaccines and effectively control many infections. We were able to completely eradicate smallpox from the world with the vaccine. Vaccines for measles, tetanus, polio, and whooping cough are saving the lives of millions of children around the world. Preventing infectious diseases through vaccines is a significant achievement of modern medical science. The idea that a vaccine for AIDS could prevent the disease seems promising. But what are the challenges in making a vaccine for AIDS? Let us see if a vaccine is possible. Due to errors in replication, all RNA viruses undergo a number of changes in their genetic structure due to errors in the course of replication. HIV is an RNA virus that changes its genome readily. In addition, there are large errors in the function of the reverse transcriptase enzyme in HIV. Therefore, there are tremendous changes in the form and function of the virus. For these reasons, it is difficult to develop an effective HIV vaccine. AIDS poses a major challenge to the social and economic systems of many developing and underdeveloped countries.

Understanding Vaccines and the Immune System:

Our immune system is the body's defence system against any microorganism that invades it. The immune system has several types of cells. Polymorphs are the cells that engulf and digest germs that enter the body. B-lymphocytes release antibodies that fight against the bacteria. CD4+-lymphocytes (T-helper cells) are cells that activate macrophages and destroy microorganisms.

The central idea of a vaccine is to make the pathogen or its components in non-harmful form and introduce them to the immune system. As a result, the vaccine properly activates the body's immune system against the pathogen. The next time the pathogen enters the person's body, it prevents infection from establishing in the body. Vaccines can prevent infection in some cases. In some cases, vaccines can reduce the severity of the disease.

We can stimulate our immune system by introducing into the body microorganisms, their components, or the toxins they release in such a way that they are not able to cause disease. The microorganism or its components are called a vaccine. The microorganisms or their components that enter through the vaccine

Live, Attenuated Vaccine
Complete germ that has been weakened.

Inactivated Vaccine
Dead version of the complete germ.

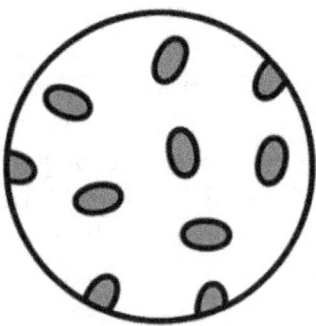

Toxoid Vaccine
Contains a toxin produced by a virus or bacteria, rather than the germ itself.

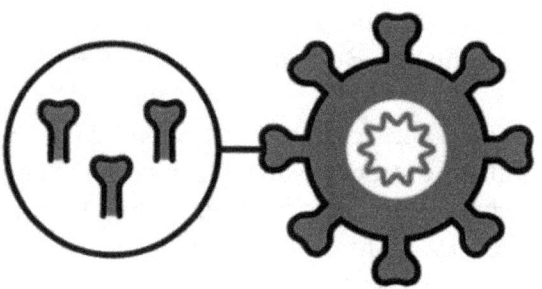

Subunit Vaccine
Contains a specific piece of the germ (like one or a few proteins).

contribute to

    the formation of antibodies and other protective cells by stimulating the immune system. These help in preventing diseases. For instance, individuals receiving a tuberculosis vaccination develop antibodies and protective cells against the disease. So, the person acquires the ability to face adversity. Vaccines are available for many diseases. In 1796, Edward Jenner introduced the first smallpox vaccine. The role of vaccines in the control of infection is unparalleled. This is a safe, simple, inexpensive, and effective method.

Various Types of Vaccines

Viral vector vaccines use a modified, harmless virus as a carrier to deliver instructions for making a specific protein from the virus we want to protect against (like SARS-CoV-2, which causes COVID-19). Our cells then produce this viral protein, and our immune system learns to recognize and fight it. The COVID-19 vaccines from AstraZeneca and Johnson & Johnson work this way.

mRNA vaccines, on the other hand, contain synthetic genetic material (mRNA) that directly instructs our cells to produce the viral protein. This mRNA is packaged in tiny, protective particles. Our immune system then learns to recognize and fight off this viral protein. The Pfizer-BioNTech and Moderna COVID-19 vaccines use this mRNA technology. Both types of vaccines do not contain live viruses, so they cannot make us sick. But they help our bodies prepare for the real virus by teaching our immune systems to recognize and attack it.

The Complexity of HIV: A Moving Target: HIV is the virus that causes AIDS. This incredibly small microbe poses significant challenges. Before developing a vaccine for any disease, the causative agent (pathogen) must be thoroughly studied. Although HIV was only discovered in 1983, scientists have learned a lot about it through ongoing research. The human immunodeficiency virus (HIV) is the most thoroughly studied microbe in human history.

Most of the vaccines we commonly use work by preventing infection altogether or significantly reducing the severity of a disease. This is true for diseases like measles, polio, and influenza. However, HIV presents a unique challenge due to its ability to integrate its genetic material into human DNA, leading to a persistent, lifelong infection. This key difference means that for HIV, our goal is a vaccine that completely prevents infection from occurring in the first place.

However, the virus can often undergo subtle changes in its genetic structure. A vaccine can only be developed against a stable form. Because the virus changes during replication, vaccines developed over many years, using one form as a model, will not work for subsequent generations. HIV can change its genetic structure by about one percent when cells divide from one generation to the next. No other organism in nature has such an immense potential for genetic changes (mutations) as HIV. To put it in perspective, in just two years, HIV can attain the level of genetic change that occurs in two million years of human evolution. This is a major hurdle in vaccine development.

HIV can take many different forms, with great genetic changes and mutations, even when it grows in a single patient. While HIV is rapidly replicating, some genetic mutations render many viral particles (virions) inactive. Furthermore, the HIV structure undergoes significant changes on a continuous basis. Because of this extreme genetic and morphological variability, it is difficult to develop a vaccine against HIV. A vaccine that targets a single standard form cannot address all these variations. We all know that influenza changes its morphology rapidly; hence, we need to develop vaccines every year. However, HIV is incorporated into the human genome and changes its genetic code to confer changes in structure that provide the ability to evade vaccines.

Hurdles in HIV Vaccine Development:

HIV can only infect humans, not animals. Similarly, HIV does not infect chimpanzees. Hence, there is no animal model candidate vaccine trial. Since AIDS is a serious and life-threatening disease, testing vaccines on humans, not animals, raises a number of ethical and human rights issues. This is a major hurdle in vaccine development research. Researchers are exploring alternative models, such as humanized mice or non-human primates infected with the simian immunodeficiency virus (SIV), which shares similarities with HIV, to study the virus and test potential vaccine candidates. In addition, HIV does not progress to AIDS until many years after infection. In 1983, when researchers isolated the human immunodeficiency virus from an AIDS patient's lymph node, they were jubilant, thinking they could develop a vaccine for the virus within two to three years. However, only a few months after the introduction of Zidovudine for HIV treatment in 1987, the mutational potential of HIV became apparent as the drug's effectiveness waned.

Diverse Forms and Global Implications:

There are two main types of HIV: HIV-1 and HIV-2. More than 95% of the world's population has HIV-1. The prevalence of HIV-2 in some countries in Africa and the Indian subcontinent is between 6% and 1%. Two types of viruses can infect the same person. In HIV-1, in the main M group, there are 9 clades of variants that show some variation. There are more than 100 circulating recombinant forms (CRFs) formed by different clades. HIV-2 also has some genetic variation. The genetic diversity of HIV is extremely high. Vaccine experiments should be carried out, taking into account all these clades. There are different clades in various parts of the world. A vaccine against one virus clade may not be able to control another. Despite all these difficulties, scientists around the world are working tirelessly to develop an AIDS vaccine.

Current Research Directions and Future Hopes:

Currently, research is underway to develop an HIV vaccine using components that do not alter the HIV envelope protein. The vaccine candidates are being evaluated for their ability to elicit broad neutralizing antibodies (bNAbs) that can block and neutralize various strains of HIV. These bNAbs are of great interest because they have the potential to neutralize a wide variety of HIV strains, making them a promising target for vaccine development efforts.

Other promising approaches include vaccines that aim to stimulate strong T-cell responses to eliminate HIV-infected cells, as well as strategies utilizing viral vectors to deliver HIV proteins and trigger an immune response against the virus.

An ideally effective HIV vaccine would provide 100% protection against HIV infection. However, achieving complete efficacy is an immense challenge. Vaccines that offer a high but not perfect level of protection can still be considered suitable for widespread use, provided their efficacy exceeds a 50% threshold. Regulatory authorities typically approve vaccines demonstrating more than 50% efficacy for widespread deployment.

While a highly effective HIV vaccine remains the ultimate goal, even a moderately effective vaccine could significantly reduce HIV transmission rates and disease burden, particularly in high-prevalence regions. A vaccine with moderate efficacy could still make a substantial impact on the HIV/AIDS pandemic.

Despite extensive research efforts and testing hundreds of HIV vaccine candidates so far, none have proven effective enough to gain regulatory approval. Due to the numerous scientific obstacles and difficulties posed by HIV's characteristics, developing an effective HIV vaccine has remained an elusive goal to date.

In long-term non-progressors / elite controllers who do not have health deterioration for a long time despite HIV infection, CD8 cells (cytotoxic T lymphocytes, or CTL) remain active and control HIV. Based on this understanding, researchers are actively working to develop a vaccine.

A small group of individuals known as long-term non-progressors, or elite controllers exhibit a unique ability to control HIV infection without experiencing significant health decline. In these individuals, CD8 T cells (cytotoxic T lymphocytes, or CTLs) remain highly active and effectively suppress HIV replication. Researchers are intensely studying this phenomenon to understand the mechanisms behind this natural control and leverage these insights to develop effective HIV vaccines and cure strategies.

Prevention Strategies and the Need for a Vaccine:

Currently, barrier methods (male and female condoms) and pre-exposure prophylaxis (PrEP) methods are widely in use for the prevention of HIV transmission. Due to some limitations in their use and the economic burden, there is a need for an effective HIV vaccine. Let us hope that in the coming years, the experiments of scientists will bear fruit and an effective HIV vaccine will be available, as vaccines are available for some diseases.

Due to inherent limitations in their use and the economic burden, there is a need for an effective HIV vaccine. Let us hope that in the coming years, the experiments of scientists will bear fruit and an effective HIV vaccine will be available, as vaccines are available for some diseases.

A Continuous Quest: The Future of HIV Vaccine Research

Despite the numerous challenges, the pursuit of an effective HIV vaccine continues with unwavering determination. Scientists remain hopeful that ongoing research and technological advancements will ultimately lead to a breakthrough, paving the way for a world free from the threat of HIV/AIDS.

20. AIDS impact on women and Children

AIDS has become a terrifying threat for women and girls due to societal discrimination and biological factors that render them vulnerable to the disease.

The Challenge of AIDS: A Disproportionate Impact

The disease known as AIDS, or acquired immunodeficiency syndrome, has a reputation for causing widespread harm, fear, and social stigma. Initially, it was believed that the illness primarily affected men who inject drugs and those who have sex with men. In most developed countries, this was largely the case. However, in developing and underdeveloped nations, the disease spreads mainly through unprotected heterosexual intercourse, which presents a significant threat to entire populations.

Social and Economic Factors: Fuelling the Epidemic

In developed nations, women and men enjoy almost equal social standing, and talking about sex is not frowned upon. This has simplified the process of raising awareness and educating people about the ways in which HIV can spread. Rich nations have successfully stopped, to the maximum extent, the spread of AIDS. Simultaneously, AIDS is spreading in developing and impoverished nations due to factors like women's marginalization, acute infrastructural shortages, poverty, illiteracy, taboos around discussing sex, and migration to metropolitan regions for work. It is challenging to increase awareness and encourage preventive measures because there are so many compelling issues.

Even if promiscuity plays a significant role in the transmission of AIDS, it is imperative to address the catalysing factors of the disease's transmission. The discussion of women's and children's rights has also gained attention because of the AIDS epidemic.

Biological and Anatomical Vulnerabilities:

Due to their inherent vulnerability, women are more likely to fall victim to AIDS in several ways. Women are more susceptible than men to getting HIV during sexual activity due to their anatomy, and the risk is increased when semen remains in the vagina for an extended period of time. Furthermore, effective transmission of the virus from men to women is facilitated by the high concentration of the virus in men's semen. Since many reproductive tract diseases in women are not immediately apparent, they may delay getting medical attention, which raises their chance of contracting HIV.

Even among healthy individuals, the risk of HIV transmission per sexual act is higher from male to female than from female to male. The probability of transmission from an HIV-positive woman to a man during a single sexual encounter is approximately 0.04% (or once in 2,380 encounters), while the probability of transmission from an HIV-positive man to a woman is around 0.08% (or once in 1,234 sexual acts). As a result, although HIV mostly affects male homosexuals and injecting drug users in wealthy nations, 54% of HIV patients globally are today female.

Socio-cultural practices and gender inequality:

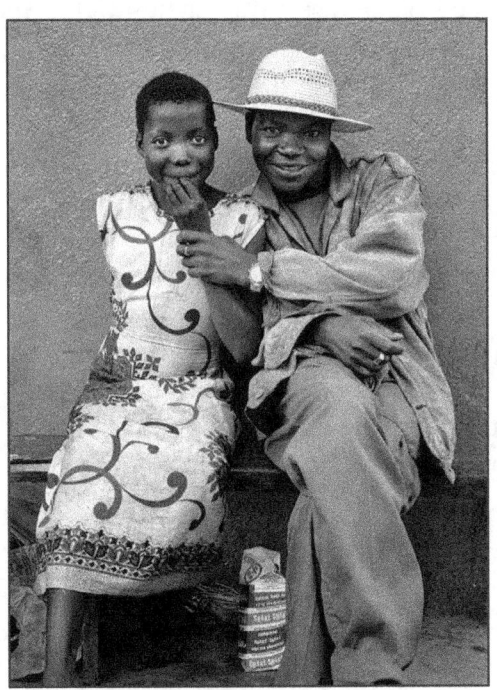

Older men having sex with younger ladies was a practice known as "sugar daddy" in various African countries. In this case, the male uses the impoverished girl for his sexual pleasure while also providing her with some financial assistance. Girls are more likely than boys to contract HIV when they are young. For this reason, women account for two-thirds (67%) of new HIV infections among Africans aged 15 to 24.

HIV is a social and natural risk that discrimination against women creates because of the double standards of many communities worldwide. Because of the false belief that having intercourse with younger girls lowers the risk of contracting diseases, the prevalence of sexual violence against women is a major concern. Some men may not feel guilty about having sex with sex workers for acquiring 'experience' in sex before getting married. They run the risk of passing it on to their spouses if they get the virus before getting married. Women and girls are exposed to AIDS at an early age following marriage due to men's premarital blunders. Some African and Asian communities marry off girls between the ages of 12 and 14.

Men are typically the ones that work and provide a livelihood for the family in underdeveloped nations. As men are financially independent, visit sex workers and other women in extramarital sex contract sexually transmitted infections. Back home, they have sex with their gullible wives and pass infections on to them. In this sense, women might become HIV positive without realizing it, even when it is not their fault. In these situations, women are financially dependent on men, making them powerless over their spouses. Even when they are ill, women are hesitant to seek medical attention for themselves. Women are thus deprived of their entitlement to healthcare.

Lack of Awareness and Education:

In some communities, girls and women may have limited awareness of issues like AIDS and STDs due to factors such as restricted access to education and information. They are consequently unable to identify the illness in its early stages and to take the appropriate safeguards.

Political Factors and Legal Barriers:

HIV infection among women is also being spread by political considerations. There are several nations that forbid organized prostitution, including India. A certain number of girls and women are forced or choose to enter this field. Such women cannot negotiate with client to use condoms. Even though these ladies are aware that using a condom helps prevent HIV and other inherited diseases, they are powerless to protect themselves. Because clients want these younger females in the hopes that they may not be HIV positive or other infections, the number of girls who are coerced into prostitution is rising. If women who commit adultery because of financial difficulties argue with their partners, men may discard them. If they resist, those who enter the profession because of oppression risk bodily harm or even death. Certain old traditional customs involving the dedication of girls and women to temples or deities, such as Devadasi, Basivi, Jogini, and Matangi, have unintentionally led to the exploitation of these individuals and their involvement in prostitution in certain areas. Women of reproductive age make up more than 90% of those living with HIV. One-third of babies delivered to HIV-positive women in underdeveloped nations will carry the infection if they do not receive treatment. After their spouses pass away from HIV, mothers in poor countries are compelled to work and force their children into prostitution.

The stark contrast in HIV prevalence between societies that empower women and those that perpetuate gender inequality is a powerful call to action. Investing in women's social and economic advancement is not only a moral imperative; it is a crucial step towards controlling the AIDS epidemic and building stronger, healthier communities.

21. HIV and Medical profession

There is a negligible risk to healthcare workers of acquiring this virus if safety measures are followed.

HIV Transmission Risk in Healthcare Settings:

While the risk of HIV transmission in healthcare settings is very low with proper precautions, it's essential for medical professionals to be aware of potential exposure and adhere to strict safety protocols. Doctors, laboratory technicians, and nursing staff often work with patients' body fluids and secretions, which can contain the virus.

Evolution of Safety Measures:

In the early days of the AIDS epidemic, when knowledge about transmission routes was limited, healthcare workers took extreme measures, sometimes wearing full protective gear akin to astronauts. Today, we understand that HIV transmission primarily occurs through direct contact with infected bodily fluids. By adhering to universal precautions, healthcare professionals can significantly minimize the risk of infection in the workplace.

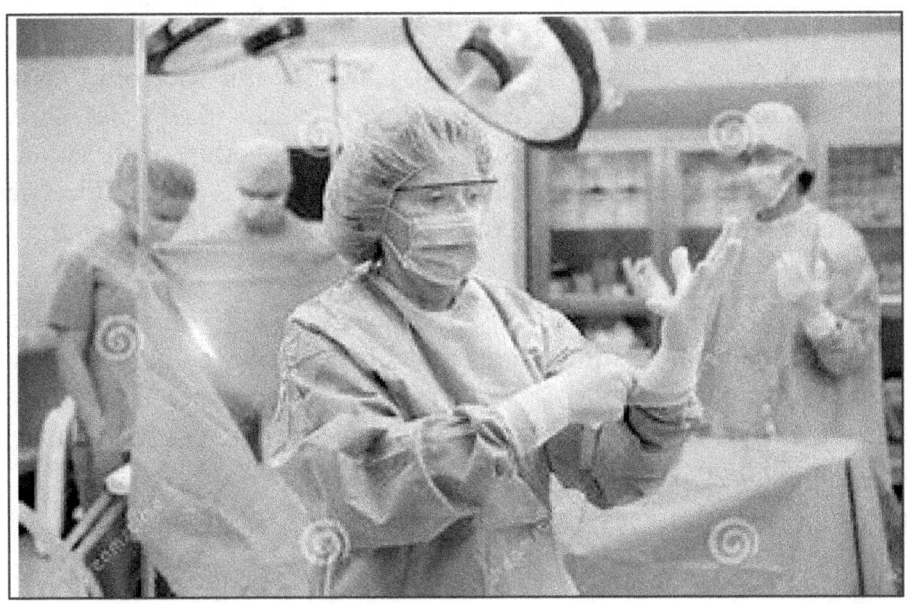

Universal Precautions: A Foundation for Safety

Universal precautions, as outlined by the US Centers for Disease Control and Prevention (CDC), require healthcare workers to avoid direct contact with bodily fluids and blood by using appropriate protective barriers. This includes wearing gloves, aprons, masks, eye protection, and gowns when necessary. Proper hand hygiene before and after patient contact is also crucial, along with the safe handling and disposal of sharp instruments like needles and scalpels. These instruments should be discarded only in designated sharps containers. Avoid recapping or bending the needles.

While HIV can be present in saliva, the risk of transmission through this route is exceedingly low. Current CPR guidelines prioritize compression-only CPR, eliminating the need for mouth-to-mouth resuscitation and further minimizing any potential risk.

Specific Precautions for Different Procedures:

Universal precautions recommend the use of gloves for all procedures involving potential contact with blood or body fluids, including administering injections or intravenous fluids. This minimizes the risk of exposure to bloodborne pathogens, including HIV. Staff with open wounds or skin conditions should avoid tasks involving potential contact with bodily fluids until healed. Additionally, blood samples collected for laboratory tests should be properly sealed to prevent spills, and all necessary precautions should be taken during testing procedures. By adhering to these guidelines, the risk of contracting HIV from patients in the medical profession is significantly reduced.

Risk of Transmission and Importance of Vigilance:

The U.S. Centers for Disease Control (CDC) reports that from 1981 to 2010, accidental needlestick injuries were the primary cause of HIV infection in 57 medical and health workers. Experts estimate the probability of infection from a single needlestick to be around 0.23%. However, it is crucial for healthcare professionals to remain vigilant and consistently adhere to universal precautions to prevent even these rare occurrences.

Blood-borne hepatitis B virus and hepatitis C pose a higher risk of transmission in healthcare settings compared to HIV. However, both hepatitis B and C are currently curable, while HIV remains a lifelong infection. This further emphasizes the importance of adhering to universal precautions to minimize the risk of exposure to all bloodborne pathogens.

Post-Exposure Prophylaxis (PEP):

In the event of an accidental needlestick or exposure to an HIV-positive patient's blood, immediate action is crucial. Allow the wound to bleed freely and rinse it thoroughly with clean water. Post-exposure prophylaxis (PEP), a two-drug combination of antiretroviral drugs, should be initiated as soon as possible after potential exposure. PEP is most effective when started immediately and taken consistently for the prescribed duration.

While the risk of HIV transmission to medical personnel is low with proper precautions, it is important to avoid complacency. The availability of PEP and adherence to universal precautions provide significant protection for healthcare workers and ensure a safe environment for both patients and professionals.

22. HIV and Skin diseases

HIV patients are more prone to skin diseases. Although almost none of these skin diseases are fatal, they may lead to depression and anxiety in patients.

Our skin is an introduction to the world. It is the largest organ in the human body, covering and protecting our bones, muscles, and internal organs. Skin encompasses nails, hair, and mucous membranes, playing a crucial role in our interaction with the environment. Despite its superficial nature, society often perceives people based on the appearance and health of their skin. It is common for people to form judgments based on external appearance and beauty.

Skin as a Barrier and its Vulnerability:

Beyond its societal implications, skin serves several essential biological functions. It acts as a barrier against harmful pathogens, UV radiation, and physical injury. The skin regulates body temperature through sweating, which helps maintain hydration levels. Additionally, the skin is rich in nerve endings, allowing us to experience sensations such as touch, pressure, and temperature.

Therefore, caring for our skin is vital not only for our appearance but also for our overall health and wellbeing. Maintaining healthy skin involves a multifaceted approach, including proper hygiene, protection, and a balanced diet. By understanding the importance of our skin and taking steps to protect it, we can ensure its optimal function and appearance.

A person's skin is the part of the body that is constantly in contact with the environment. Nature constantly exposes the skin to a variety of microorganisms in the air. Many microorganisms in the environment do not harm us in any way. Certain microorganisms, however, can cause diseases. Generally, animals and plants that are somewhat weak are susceptible to microbial diseases. Skin plays the first and foremost role in protecting humans from adverse environmental conditions and harmful germs. Otherwise, humans would have become extinct among many harmful microorganisms.

Skin Conditions in HIV/AIDS:

Kaposi's sarcoma, a skin cancer, is the only skin condition in the AIDS definition. Kaposi's sarcoma is an AIDS-defining illness because it often indicates a severely weakened immune system, making individuals more susceptible to this type of cancer. These are some other conditions that indicate damaged immunity: Molluscum contagiosum, severe recurrent herpes simplex virus infections, and herpes zoster. Although some skin diseases are not life-threatening, they can have profound consequences. Kaposi sarcoma is common in Africa and the Americas. But it is rare in many Asian countries, including India.

Social Stigma and Quality of Life:

Skin diseases often carry a social stigma, as they can affect a person's appearance and lead to feelings of self-consciousness, shame, or even discrimination. This is one reason individuals may prioritize the treatment of skin conditions over other, potentially more serious health issues. The visible nature of skin diseases can significantly impact a person's quality of life and mental well-being.

In people living with HIV, the gradual weakening of the immune system makes them more susceptible to various infections, including those affecting the skin. This vulnerability increases the risk of developing skin problems caused by parasites, bacteria, viruses, and fungi. While skin diseases are relatively rare in developed countries due to better hygiene and access to healthcare, they are much more prevalent in developing regions. Factors such as poor sanitation, crowded living conditions, and a higher prevalence of disease-carrying insects contribute to this disparity. As a result, HIV patients in these countries often experience a range of skin conditions, including hives, abscesses, warts, psoriasis, severe itching, extensive ringworm (tinea), nail damage, and allergies. Although these conditions may not be life-threatening, they can significantly impact a patient's quality of life and contribute to feelings of stigma and distress.

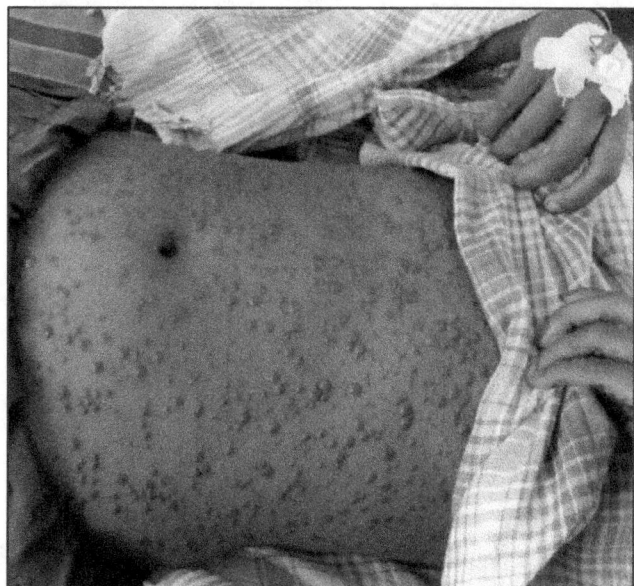

The weakened immune system in HIV patients allows skin diseases to spread and progress rapidly, often presenting with atypical or exaggerated symptoms. This can make diagnosis challenging for healthcare providers, potentially leading to delays or misdiagnosis.

FA 15-year-old, infected with HIV at birth presented with a viral skin disease resembling the now-extinct smallpox.

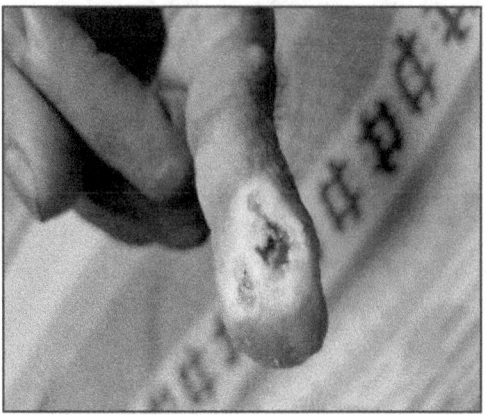 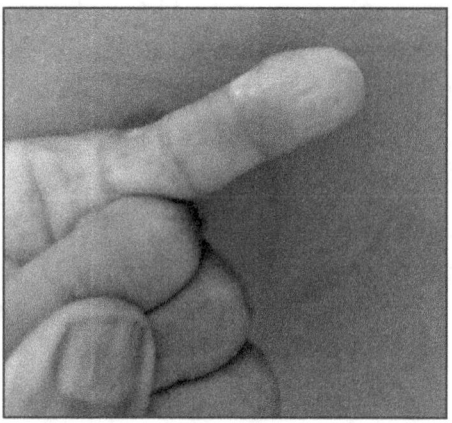

A 45-year-old HIV patient, who works as an agriculturist, developed a worsening finger ulcer despite two months of various treatments. Healed completely in 15 days with appropriate treatment'

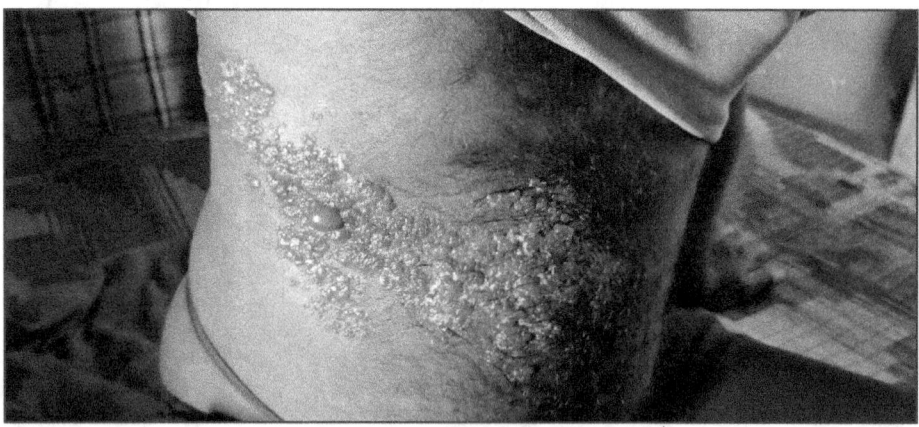

Although this disease can manifest with varying severity, its atypical presentation in HIV patients often necessitates diagnosis by highly experienced doctors.

23. UNAIDS and other Global organizations' fight against AIDS

With decades of effort on the part of the World Health Organization, UNAIDS, and other agencies, the devastating effects of AIDS could be reduced.

The World Health Organization, UNAIDS, and all member countries have fought the decades-long AIDS epidemic in extraordinary ways that have largely stopped the devastation and tragedy.

Early Initiatives: The WHO's Global Program on AIDS

Recognizing that AIDS was becoming a major global problem, the World Health Organization launched the Global Program to Fight AIDS on February 1, 1987. Dr. Jonathan Mann, who championed AIDS as a human rights issue, became the first director of the department, which has been successful in preparing world leaders and people to fight AIDS. AIDS victims and international distribution companies were involved in a big way. The International Council for AIDS Service Organizations (ICASO) promoted the creation of the Global Network of Positive People (GNP+) organizations. The World Health Organization has been celebrating World AIDS Day since December 1, 1988, to raise public awareness of AIDS and show solidarity with AIDS victims.

UNAIDS and Collaborative Efforts:

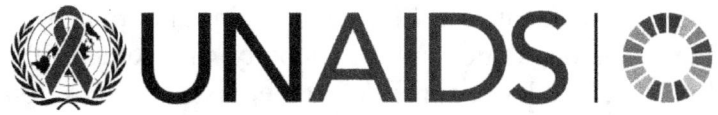

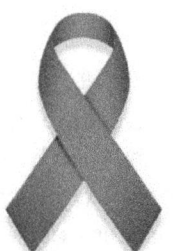

On January 1, 1996, the United Nations launched UNAIDS (The Joint United Nations Programme on HIV/AIDS) with 11 co-sponsoring organizations. Every year, UNAIDS provides a theme for countries to use in observing World AIDS Day. The UNAIDS logo incorporates elements that symbolize the organization's commitment to addressing HIV/AIDS as part of the broader Sustainable Development Goals.

Expanding Access: PEPFAR and the Global Fund

In 2003, President George W. Bush launched the 'President's Emergency Plan for AIDS Relief,' a program to make AIDS treatment available to patients in poor countries. This program has saved 25 million lives in 20 years. Estimates indicate that the program, currently implemented in over 50 countries, contributed to a 2.1 percent increase in GDP growth in those countries from 2004 to 2018. Launched in 2002, the Global Fund to Fight AIDS, Tuberculosis, and Malaria (The Global Fund) has made significant achievements in addressing these diseases through large-scale fundraising.

Beyond the Major Players: A Diverse Landscape of Support

While the World Health Organization, UNAIDS, and the Global Fund play central roles in the global response to HIV/AIDS, numerous other organizations contribute significantly to this ongoing fight. The U.S. President's Emergency Plan for AIDS Relief (PEPFAR) has been instrumental in providing life-saving treatment and prevention services in many countries, particularly in Africa. Unitaid focuses on increasing access to affordable medications and diagnostics for HIV/AIDS, tuberculosis, and malaria, while Médecins Sans Frontières (MSF) delivers crucial care in resource-limited settings and conflict zones. The International AIDS Society (IAS) advances research, treatment, and care through its vast network of professionals and advocates.

Beyond these international actors, countless local and regional organizations play vital roles within their communities. Grassroots efforts are essential for reaching marginalized populations, providing culturally appropriate services, and advocating for the needs of people living with HIV/AIDS. These organizations often work on the frontlines, delivering prevention education, testing services, and support programs, and their contributions are invaluable in the fight against the epidemic.

Sex is one of the basic instincts of life, and it begins after puberty. Every year, a certain percentage of the population reaches puberty, and some of them become sexually active. However, this does not mean that there is no need to stop the spread of HIV. Awareness campaigns should sustain uninterrupted because, due to indifference, those who were previously unaware of HIV are at risk of contracting the disease.

Community Engagement: Leading the Charge

Since 1988, World AIDS Day has been observed globally on December 1 to show solidarity with the victims of AIDS, to pay tribute to the victims of AIDS, to inspire people, and to honour the work of NGOs and medical personnel working in this field. Since 1991, the Red Ribbon has been used to raise awareness of AIDS (and for drug abuse, drunk driving, and multiple sclerosis).

HIV-AIDS

The theme of World AIDS Day 2023 is 'Let Communities Lead'. UNAIDS calls on people living with AIDS, victims of AIDS who have lost their loved ones, those at risk of HIV, and those belonging to these groups to lead from the front in creating awareness about AIDS.

24. Indian Generics and Global HIV Treatment Equity

A Crisis of Access: The HIV/AIDS Treatment Gap

The Indian pharmaceutical industry has played a pivotal role in making life-saving antiretroviral (ARV) drugs accessible and affordable for millions of people living with HIV/AIDS worldwide. This remarkable achievement has its roots in the early 2000s, when the global AIDS crisis was at its peak and the prohibitive costs of patented ARV medications made them inaccessible to a vast majority of patients, particularly in low- and middle-income countries.

A Child's Plea: Nkosi Johnson and the Call to Action

In a landmark speech at the 13th International AIDS Conference in Durban, South Africa, in 2000, a young South African boy named Nkosi Johnson, who was born with HIV, delivered a powerful and emotional plea that resonated across the globe. At the tender age of 11, Nkosi's words resonated with the struggles faced by countless individuals living with HIV/AIDS, and his message struck a chord with the Indian pharmaceutical industry.

India's Response: Stepping Up to the Challenge

Indian companies, both domestic and multinational corporations (MNCs) operating within the country, recognized the urgent need to address this crisis. Leveraging India's expertise in generic drug manufacturing and a favourable legal framework that allowed the production of affordable generic versions of patented drugs, these companies stepped up to the challenge.

A Collective Effort: Indian Companies Join the Cause

One of the key players in this endeavour was Cipla, an Indian pharmaceutical giant. In 2001, Cipla made headlines by offering a triple-drug combination ARV for less than $1 per day, a fraction of the cost charged by major pharmaceutical companies at the time. This bold move shook the industry and paved the way for other Indian companies to follow suit.

Companies like Aurobindo Pharma, Hetero Drugs, Mylan (now Viatris), Emcure, Laurus Labs, Macleods Pharmaceuticals, Natco Pharma, Alkem Laboratories, Biomatrix Biotech, and Strides Pharma, among others, joined the effort, leveraging their manufacturing capabilities and economies of scale to produce high-quality generic ARVs at affordable prices. These efforts were further bolstered by the Indian government's decision to grant compulsory licenses, allowing domestic companies to manufacture patented drugs without the consent of the patent holders, in the interest of public health.

Impact and Reach: Transforming the Global Picture

The impact of these efforts was far-reaching. Indian generic ARVs not only made treatment accessible to millions within the country but also facilitated the rapid scale-up of HIV/AIDS treatment programs in various African and other resource-limited nations. Organizations like the Clinton Health Access Initiative (CHAI) and the Global Fund to Fight AIDS, Tuberculosis, and Malaria played crucial roles in procuring and distributing these affordable ARVs worldwide.

Nkosi Johnson's speech at the 13th International AIDS Conference served as a powerful catalyst, igniting a movement within the Indian pharmaceutical industry to prioritize access to affordable healthcare over profit margins. The industry's response to this call to action has been instrumental in transforming the global HIV/AIDS landscape, saving millions of lives, and giving hope to countless individuals affected by this devastating disease.

Today, the Indian pharmaceutical industry continues to be a vital player in the global fight against HIV/AIDS, supplying more than 80% of the world's generic ARV medications. This commitment to making essential medicines accessible and affordable has solidified India's reputation as the "pharmacy of the world," and the industry's efforts have set a precedent for addressing other public health challenges through innovative and compassionate approaches.

Innovator Pharma Reshaping the HIV/AIDS Landscape

While the Indian pharmaceutical industry played a critical role in making ARVs affordable and accessible, it is essential to acknowledge the contributions of innovator companies, primarily multinational pharmaceutical corporations, in developing these life-saving drugs. Companies like GlaxoSmithKline, Gilead Sciences, Bristol-Myers Squibb, Merck & Co., and ViiV Healthcare (a joint venture between GlaxoSmithKline, Pfizer, and Shionogi) have been at the forefront of research and development, investing substantial resources into discovering and developing groundbreaking ARV medications. Their scientific breakthroughs and rigorous clinical trials paved the way for the treatment options available today, and their ongoing research efforts continue to push the boundaries of HIV/AIDS treatment and prevention.

Bridging the Gap: Bringing ARVs to Developing Nations

The Medicines Patent Pool (MPP) is a United Nations-backed organization that works to increase access to affordable HIV, hepatitis, and tuberculosis treatments in developing countries. It negotiates with patent holders to license their intellectual property to generic manufacturers in exchange for royalties. Since 2010, MPP has signed agreements for 13 HIV antiretroviral drugs and one technology, enabling generic production in 135 countries. This has provided over 22 million patient-years of HIV treatment as of 2022. MPP's work has been pivotal for the

Indian generic drug industry to manufacture low-cost ARV versions. Its licensing allows Indian companies like Cipla and Aurobindo to legally produce generics while paying royalties. This increased competition has reduced prices by 73.5% for certain HIV regimens in developing nations. MPP aims to ensure sustainable supplies through quality standards and public reporting requirements.

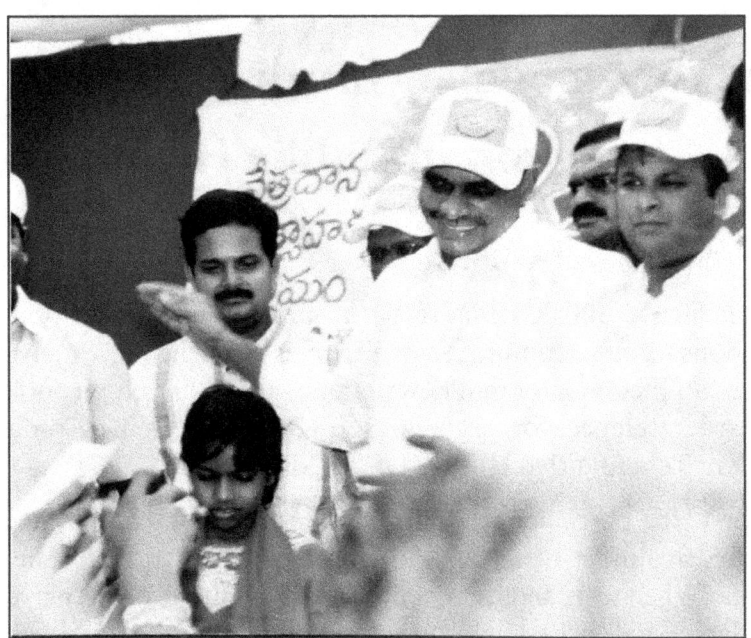

On July 4, 2005, Dr Yanamadala participated in the launch of the AIDS campaign 'ASHA' at Palakollu with Chief Minister Dr. YS Rajasekhara Reddy. Lav Agarwal, the then-Collector and later Joint Secretary of the Union Health Ministry, also in the picture.

Dr. Yanamadala Murali Krishna: A Champion in Public Health

Addressing the Challenges of AIDS:

Dr. Yanamadala Murali Krishna raised awareness of AIDS among Telugu-speaking populations through comprehensive articles published in widely read daily newspapers and adult literacy program newsletters. His 2000 Telugu book on AIDS became a standard reference for organizers of AIDS awareness programs. He published a book in Telugu, titled HIV-AIDS, in March 2024.

He is the first HIV physician in Andhra Pradesh, India, who started a clinic in 2000. When AIDS treatment was prohibitively expensive for many, he opened a clinic in Kakinada. When tests and treatment were prohibitively expensive, he made treatment affordable and accessible by employing his clinical expertise and thorough understanding of the disease. To date, he has treated more than 6,000 HIV patients, and these patients are able to lead productive lives, support their families, and contribute to their communities.

Dr. Yanamadala's maiden research proposing a low-cost severity assessment test for HIV-TB stood out as one of 25 impactful works out of 5000 abstracts presented to the XIII International AIDS Conference in Durban, South Africa, in July 2000.

In September and October 2022, respectively, the U.S. and European AIDS treatment guidelines included his proclamation of two-drug therapy for HIV as an option, demonstrating his pioneering work.

Working in the Field of COVID-19:

Recognizing the need for a comprehensive homecare kit for mild COVID-19 that addressed the key aspects of its pathophysiology—inflammation, clotting, and secondary bacterial infections—Dr. Yanamadala developed a tailored approach. His affordable and effective homecare kit, combining Aspirin, Prednisolone, and Azithromycin to address inflammation, clotting, and potential secondary infections, saw widespread adoption in the Telugu States after its introduction in April 2021, likely saving numerous lives during the Delta variant surge.

His autobiographical medical science book, 'COVID AIDS and Me,' was published in Telugu in January 2022.

Protecting Hearts After COVID-19:

Dr. Yanamadala Murali Krishna recognized the elevated risk of heart attacks among individuals who had survived COVID-19 and alerted the public about this potential complication. He has actively championed the use of Aspirin as a preventive measure against post-COVID heart attacks, standard preventive strategy for those who have recovered from COVID-19.

Book Review

HIV-AIDS in India & Developing Countries
by Dr. Yanamadala Murali Krishna, MD,
4-50, Main Road, Indrapalem, Kakinada 533006,
Andhra Pradesh, India,
e-mail : peopleagainstaids@yahoo.co.in.
First Published : May, 2024, Pages iv + vi + 122,
Price : Rs.155.00, Outside India : US$ 7.99.

Overview :

Dr. Yanamadala Murali Krishna's HIV-AIDS in India & Developing Countries offers an in-depth, authoritative examination of the HIV-AIDS epidemic, with a particular focus on the Indian subcontinent and other developing nations. The book carefully traces the origins, transmission, and global ramifications of the HIV virus while addressing the specific socio-economic challenges faced by these regions in combating the disease. Divided into comprehensive chapters, it delves into the medical, social, and political dimensions of HIV-AIDS and provides a roadmap for both understanding the disease and implementing effective interventions.

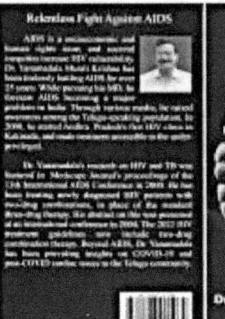
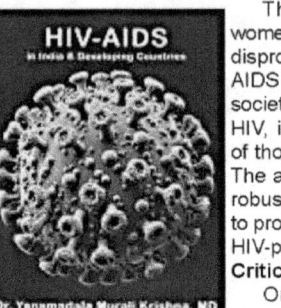

Book Structure and Content :

The book begins with a historical account of the origins of HIV, followed by a detailed exploration of the global impact of the disease, as highlighted in the early chapters. Chapters 1 to 4 set the stage by exploring the epidemiology and biological mechanisms of the virus, offering a global perspective on the HIV pandemic. Dr. Krishna's writing style is clear, concise, and devoid of unnecessary medical jargon, making it accessible to a wider audience, including policymakers, healthcare workers, and public health students.

One of the most compelling aspects of the book is the chapter on HIV-AIDS in India, where Dr. Krishna examines the unique trajectory of the disease within the subcontinent. This section not only emphasizes the high-risk groups and cultural factors influencing the spread of the disease but also highlights the significant progress India has made through its generics industry and global contributions to HIV treatment equity.

The author places great emphasis on prevention strategies and treatment protocols, particularly the section on Two-Drug Antiretroviral Therapy, which is a crucial read for healthcare professionals in resource-limited settings. In the Indian context, the narrative successfully addresses the cultural stigmatization of the disease and the lack of adequate healthcare infrastructure, making a strong case for global collaboration in both prevention and treatment efforts.

Highlights :

The chapters on HIV and Tuberculosis, HIV and Pregnancy, and the role of UNAIDS in coordinating a global response to AIDS are particularly noteworthy. Dr. Krishna carefully analyzes the co-infection of HIV and TB, an urgent issue in India and other developing nations, and outlines diagnostic approaches like the Tuberculin Response for better management of HIV-TB patients.

Moreover, the book dedicates a thoughtful chapter to HIV Cure Research and the promise of an AIDS vaccine, discussing the scientific, financial, and ethical challenges of vaccine development. The reader gains valuable insight into the global fight against AIDS, emphasizing how innovations in HIV treatment, including generic drug production in India, have substantially contributed to making antiretroviral therapy accessible to low-income countries.

The final chapters focus on women and children, a segment disproportionately affected by the AIDS epidemic, and explore the societal implications of living with HIV, including the fight for rights of those affected by the disease. The author advocates for a more robust legal and social framework to protect the rights and dignity of HIV-positive individuals.

Critical Evaluation :

One of the book's greatest strengths lies in its ability to weave together scientific information with real-world applications. Dr. Krishna's deep understanding of the epidemiological and clinical aspects of HIV-AIDS is evident throughout, as is his concern for the socio-economic contexts that hinder effective treatment in developing countries. The section on Indian generics and global HIV treatment equity presents a balanced view of the complex global pharmaceutical landscape and India's critical role in ensuring access to life-saving medications at an affordable cost.

However, while the book is comprehensive in scope, it occasionally assumes a level of pre-existing knowledge that may alienate non-specialist readers. A more detailed glossary of medical terms or an expanded introduction to antiretroviral therapies could enhance accessibility for a broader audience.

Conclusion :

HIV-AIDS in India & Developing Countries is a meticulously researched and thoughtfully presented work that offers valuable insights into one of the most critical global health challenges of our time. Dr. Yanamadala Murali Krishna's book is not only a significant academic contribution but also an essential guide for policymakers and healthcare professionals involved in the global fight against HIV. Its particular emphasis on India and other developing nations fills a crucial gap in HIV literature, making it a must-read for anyone interested in global public health.

Dr. Shambo S. Samajdar
MD DM (Clinical Pharmacology)
FIPS, Fellow Diabetes India, Fellowship Respiratory and Critical Care (WBUHS)
PG Dip Endo & Diabetes (RCP), Dip Allergy Asthma Immunology (AAAAI)
Consultant, Diabetes and Allergy-Asthma Therapeutics Specialty Clinic, Kolkata
Faculty, JMN Medical College and Hospital, Nadia

Further reading

1. The Origins of AIDS by Jacques Pepin

2. HIV Essentials by Paul E. Sax, Calvin J. Cohen, and Daniel R. Kuritzkes

3. AIDS Therapy by Raphael Dolin, Henry Masur, and Michael S. Saag

4. Principles of Virology, by Jane Flint, Vincent R. Racaniello, Glenn F. Rall, Theodora Hatziioannou, Anna Marie

5. HIV 2023/24 by Christian Hoffman and Jürgen Rockstroh

6. How to Survive a Plague: The Inside Story of How Citizens and Science Tamed AIDS by David France

7. Fundamentals of HIV Medicine by the American Academy of HIV Medicine, published by Oxford

8. Bartletts's Medical Management of HIV Infection by John G. Bartlett, Robert R. Redfield, and Paul A. Pham

9. Tropical Diseases, by Yann A. Meunier

10. UNAIDS and WHO Websites

11 Comprehensive Textbook of Infectious Diseases by MI Sahadulla and Sayenna A. Uduman

12. Microbiology Lippincott Illustrated Review by Cynthia Nau Cornelissen & Marcia Metzgar Hobbs and Sumathi Muralidhar & Suchitra Shenoy,

13. Relevant content from the websites of agencies working in the field of HIV/AIDS

14. https://en.wikipidia.org.in/index.php/Yanamadala_Murali_Krishna

KASTURI VIJAYAM

www.kasturivijayam.com
+91 9515054998

SUPPORTS

- PUBLISH YOUR BOOK AS YOUR OWN PUBLISHER.

- PAPERBACK & E-BOOK SELF-PUBLISHING

- SUPPORT PRINT ON-DEMAND.

- YOUR PRINTED BOOKS AVAILABLE AROUND THE WORLD.

- EASY TO MANAGE YOUR BOOK'S LOGISTICS AND TRACK YOUR REPORTING.

www.ingramcontent.com/pod-product-compliance
Lightning Source LLC
LaVergne TN
LVHW081543070526
838199LV00057B/3757